ADVANCED NURSING PRACTICE

ADVANCED NURSING PRACTICE

The Expanding Role of the Nurse Practitioner

CAROLE MACKAVEY, Editor

University of Texas Health Science Center—Houston Texas

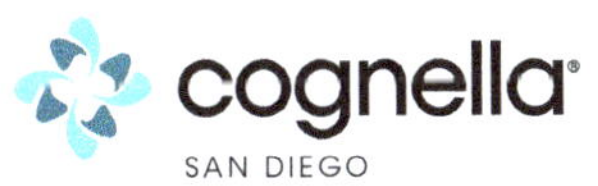

Bassim Hamadeh, CEO and Publisher
Amanda Martin, Publisher
Amy Smith, Senior Project Editor
Casey Hands, Production Editor
Jess Estrella, Senior Graphic Designer
Kara Tatum, Licensing Coordinator
Natalie Piccotti, Director of Marketing
Kassie Graves, Senior Vice President, Editorial

Printed in the United States of America.

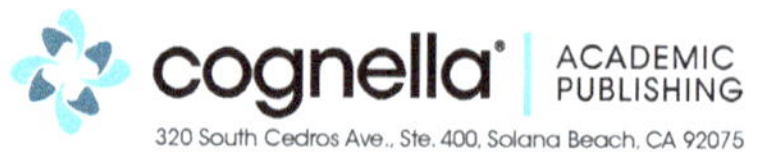

BRIEF CONTENTS

Preface xv

Reviewers xvii

Chapter 1 The Developing Role of Advanced Practice Nursing in the United States and Globally 1

Carole Mackavey

Chapter 2 Advanced Practice Nursing Education Pathway: MSN and BSN to DNP 29

Carole Mackavey and Linda Cole

Chapter 3 AACN Competencies in Advanced Practice Nursing Education and Role 47

Carole Mackavey

Chapter 4 Simulation in Advanced Practice Nursing 59

Mandi Lyons and Padma Ramaswamy

Chapter 5 Advanced Practice Nursing's Role in Social Determinants of Health 103

Kelly Kearney and Carole Mackavey

Chapter 6 Advanced Practice Nursing and Telehealth 121

Carole Mackavey

Chapter 7 APRNs in Leadership and Project Management 141

Linda Cole and Lisa Boss

Chapter 8 Health Policy and Advocacy: What Can Advanced Practice Nurses Do? 161

Kathleen Siders, Robert Carl Coghlan III, and Aastha Krebs

Chapter 9 Legal Parameters of Care and Practice 197

Kathleen Siders, Robert Coghlan III, and Aastha Krebs

Chapter 10 Transitioning From Registered Nurse to Advanced Practice Nurse/Nurse Practitioner 215

Carole Mackavey and Tammy Stout

Index 231

About the Editor 241

About the Contributors 243

DETAILED CONTENTS

Preface xv

Reviewers xvii

Chapter 1 The Developing Role of Advanced Practice Nursing in the United States and Globally 1

Carole Mackavey

Objectives 1

Questions/Challenges 1

Introduction 2

Pieces of APN History: Changing Times 2

- Resistance 3
- Nurse Practitioners 5
- History of Nursing Response to a Crisis 5
- The COVID-19 Pandemic: The Impact on Advanced Nursing Practice 7
- NP Practice 7
- CRNA-Certified Registers Nurse Anesthetist 10
- Other Changes in Practice 11

International Practice 12

- Australia 13
- Canada 14
- China 15
- The Netherlands 16
- Republic of Ireland 17
- The United Kingdom: England, Scotland, Wales, and Northern Ireland 18

Chapter Summary 20

Key Points 21

Activities 21

References 22

Chapter 2 Advanced Practice Nursing Education Pathway: MSN and BSN to DNP 29

Carole Mackavey and Linda Cole

Objectives 29
Questions/Challenges 29
Introduction 30
The Move Toward Doctoral Education 31
Challenges Faced by the DNP 32
Clinical Role of the Advanced Practice Nurse/NP 33
NP Specialty Advanced Practice Roles 34
- Nurse Educators 34
- NP Nurse Executive Leadership 35
- NP Nursing Informatics 36
- Certified Nurse–Midwives (CNM) and Women's Health Nurse Practitioners 37
- Women Health Nurse Practitioners (WHNP) 37
- Clinical Nurse Specialists (CNS) 37
- Certified Registered Nurse Anesthetists (CRNA) 39

Recent Pandemics' Impact on NP Education 40
Chapter Summary 41
Key Points 42
Activities 42
References 42

Chapter 3 AACN Competencies in Advanced Practice Nursing Education and Role 47

Carole Mackavey

Objectives 47
Questions/Challenges 47
Introduction 48
Competency in Education and Practice 48
What Is Competency-Based Education (CBE) 48
- Why Competency? 49
- Competency-Based Clinical Education 53

Chapter Summary 54
Key Points 55

Activities 55
References 55

Chapter 4 Simulation in Advanced Practice Nursing 59

Mandi Lyons and Padma Ramaswamy

Objectives 59
Questions/Challenges 60
Introduction 60
Historical Foundations of Simulation 61
Evolution of Simulation in Nursing 63
Simulation: Enhancing Education and Practice 67
  Prelicensure Nursing Programs 68
  Advanced Practice Nursing Programs 69
  Continued Professional Development 72
Theoretical Frameworks 73
  Kolb's Experiential Learning Theory 73
  Knowles' Adult Learning Theory 74
  The Reflective Practitioner Theory 74
Benefits and Limitations of Simulation in Nursing 75
Navigating Simulation 78
  Classification of Simulation 78
  Simulation Modalities 79
Utilizing Simulated Participants 81
Methods 83
Designing Simulation: What to Consider 84
Simulation Phases: Prebriefing, Design, and Debriefing 86
  Prebriefing 86
  Simulation Design 89
  Debriefing 89
Evaluation in Simulation 92
  Formative Evaluation 92
  Summative Evaluation 93
  High-Stakes Evaluation 93
Evaluation Tools 94
Moving Forward With Simulation in Advanced Practice Nursing Education 94

Chapter Summary 95
Key Points 96
Activities 97
References 97

Chapter 5 Advanced Practice Nursing's Role in Social Determinants of Health 103

Kelly Kearney and Carole Mackavey

Objectives 103
Questions/Challenges 103
Introduction: What Are the Social Determinants of Health 104
Vulnerable Populations: Who Are the Vulnerable Populations? 107
Health Disparity vs. Health Equity 108
 What Is Health Disparity? 108
 So What Is Health Equity? 110
Advanced Practice Role in Caring for Vulnerable Populations 113
Impacts of SDOHs on Mental Health 114
Impacts of SDOHs on Rural Health Care 115
Chapter Summary 116
Key Points 117
Activities 117
References 117

Chapter 6 Advanced Practice Nursing and Telehealth 121

Carole Mackavey

Objectives 121
Questions/Challenges 121
Introduction 122
Defining Telehealth and Telemedicine 122
Types of Telehealth Defined 126
Telehealth Competencies 127
Advantages and Disadvantages of Telehealth 128
 Disadvantages 130
APN Practice 131
Licensure and Credentialing 131
Reimbursement Policies 131

Remaining Barriers 135
Additional Resources 135
Chapter Summary 135
Key Points 136
Activities 136
References 137

Chapter 7 APRNs in Leadership and Project Management 141

Linda Cole and Lisa Boss

Objectives 141
Questions/Challenges 141
Introduction 141
Organizational Culture 143
Leveraging Influence and Leading Teams 145
Conclusion 146
Project Management 146
- What Is Project Management? 146
- Foundational PM Principles 147
- Performance Domains 148
- Conclusion 156

Chapter Summary 156
Key Points 157
Activities 157
References 158

Chapter 8 Health Policy and Advocacy: What Can Advanced Practice Nurses Do? 161

Kathleen Siders, Robert Carl Coghlan III, and Aastha Krebs

Objectives 161
Questions/Challenges 161
Introduction 161
Policy Definitions 162
Policy Change 163
How Policy Impacts Health Care 164
Advocating for Change 170

Access to Health Care 171
Consumer Protection Provisions 173
Obtaining and Renewing Health Insurance 174
Health Insurance Cost and Variations 175
Transparency 175
Post-Introduction Analysis 176
Funding, Cost Containment Measures, and Impact on Health Care Costs 178
Cost-Containment: Medicare 179
Cost-Containment: Medicaid 180
Health Care Policy and COVID-19 181
Chapter Summary 184
Key Points 186
Activities 187
References 189

Chapter 9 Legal Parameters of Care and Practice 197

Kathleen Siders, Robert Coghlan III, and Aastha Krebs

Objectives 197
Questions/Challenges 197
Introduction 198
Practice Act 198
Consensus Model 204
Levels of Supervision in the United States 205
Health Care, Law, and Ethics 208
Chapter Summary 211
Key Points 211
Activities 212
References 213

Chapter 10 Transitioning From Registered Nurse to Advanced Practice Nurse/Nurse Practitioner 215

Carole Mackavey and Tammy Stout

Objectives 215
Questions/Challenges 215
Introduction 216

Role Transition 221
Communication: Difficult Conversations 222
Functioning as a Member of the Health Care Team 224
Patient-Centered Care 224
Chapter Summary 226
Key Points 226
Activities 227
References 227

Index 231
About the Editor 241
About the Contributors 243

PREFACE

The global turmoil caused by the COVID-19 pandemic has led to profound and lasting change within the nursing field. As healthcare systems struggled with extraordinary challenges, nurse practitioners emerged as integral team members, showing adaptability and resilience. *Advanced Nursing Practice: The Expanding Role of the Nurse Practitioner* takes a slightly different approach by examining nurse practitioners' enhanced responsibilities, skills, and contributions rather than the historical challenges. Advanced practice nursing and the nurse practitioner role are constantly evolving to meet the needs of the health care system, making them key players in shaping the future of health care.

This book explores the expanding role of the nurse practitioner, offering students insight into the changing healthcare landscape. It illustrates the nurse practitioner's adaptability in response to challenges and their critical role in advancing health care. Innovations and new technology have increased access to care, enhanced the care provided, and opened up many possibilities to be explored within the role.

Advanced Nursing Practice: The Expanding Role of the Nurse Practitioner also features pedagogical aids aimed at enhancing the learning experience and catering to diverse learning needs. These include discussion questions, student challenges, "food for thought" boxes, and student activities highlighted in each chapter. It is the authors' hope that this book will promote active learning and stimulate reflection and the spirit of inquiry.

REVIEWERS

Lisa Quinn, PhD, CRNP, MSN
Gannon University

Laree J. Schoolmeesters, PhD, RN, CNL
Queens University of Charlotte

Melody D. Randle, DNP, FNP-C, CNE
Wilmington University

CHAPTER 1

The Developing Role of Advanced Practice Nursing in the United States and Globally

Carole Mackavey

> *"I was well aware of the unmet health needs of people of all ages in the community and confident that nurses could be prepared to meet those needs by facilitating access and promoting continuity and coordination of care."*
>
> —*(Ford, 1979, p. 517)*

OBJECTIVES

Upon completion of the chapter, the student will be able to

1. examine the global expansion of advanced practice nursing
2. assess the impact of advanced practice nursing on health outcomes
3. discuss the global framework for advanced practice nursing development

QUESTIONS/CHALLENGES

1. How would you go about making a change toward independent practice?

INTRODUCTION

You might be wondering, "Why review advanced nursing practice history?" History helps us examine and understand how complex questions and dilemmas were addressed—what worked and what did not work. The first nursing practitioner training programs emerged during the 1960s, when the fight for civil rights transformed the health care landscape. Many elderly people were without insurance, and the government programs were for the "deserving Americans," such as veterans and federal employees. Social class and race were not even given much thought (Stevens, 1996).

In 1962, Michael Harrington wrote that "Another America" was 40 to 50 million poor citizens who lacked adequate medical care and were "socially invisible" to most of the population. Political upheaval and civil rights rallies stimulated politicians to support Medicare. On July 30, 1965, President Lyndon B. Johnson signed the Medicare and Medicaid Act, also known as the Social Security Amendments of 1965, into law. It established Medicare, a health insurance program for the elderly, and Medicaid, a health insurance program for people with limited income (National Archives, n.d.). At the end of World War II, there were profound changes in medical education. The military recognized special expertise physicians and offered them a higher rank and increased pay, resulting in a shift from general practice to specialty (Dalen et al., 2017). With the physician specialization underway, there was an increasing number of unfilled gaps in primary care.

PIECES OF APN HISTORY: CHANGING TIMES

In the early 1960s, Dr. Lorretta Ford, a public health nurse in Boulder, Colorado, took note of the disparities, the community's shortage of primary care physicians, and the limited health care for children and families. Dr. Ford felt nurses could fill the gap left by physician specialization with some extra training. So in 1965,

Dr. Ford and her colleague Dr. Henry K. Silver, a pediatrician at the University of Colorado Medical Center, started the first pediatric nurse practitioner (NP) model and training program. The program focused on clinical care and research on the impact of the social determinants of health. The early work of Dr. Ford, who is also the founding dean of the University of Rochester School of Nursing and the author of over 200 publications (Berg, 2020), pushed us to expand the advanced practice nursing (APN) role, form organizations, and advance our scope of practice one step at a time.

Resistance

When Dr. Ford and other early advocates of NP programs first began development, they encountered resistance. Many established health care providers believed this was not their place—the pioneers of NP. Programs had to unite and struggle to overcome these obstacles. Berg (2020) interviewed the following NP pioneers about the pushback they experienced:

- **Dr. Loretta C. Ford:** Established, tenured, and politically powerful faculty were dead set against the NP role idea and created barriers, used bullying tactics, and used isolation to try to impede the progress of the role. The question of the new role was even questioned by nursing and they asked whether or not it was even legal.
- **Dr. Deborah Kiley:** Dr. Kiley was asked, "Who do you think you are?" and was told that "nurses have no business doing doctor work."
- **Ms. Judith Lynch:** Pushback was immediate and, unfortunately, from my nursing colleagues. My biggest challenge was with the state of New York. In the 1970s, the attorney general refused to legally recognize NPs, even though the State Department of Health hired NPs. The Nurse Practice Act covered NP practice but not prescriptive authority. She was threatened with legal

action. As a result, she became politically active with the New York State Nurses Association and helped create an NP act that allowed NPs to practice legally.

- **Mr. Richard Meadows:** His chief nursing officer (CNO) called him a "prima donna," and the physician said his patients would not see an NP.
- **Dr. Barbara Sheer:** The issues that hindered practice involved major retail pharmacy chains deciding not to honor NP prescriptions. They used cosigned prescriptions and called in prescriptions, and finally, the Pennsylvania Rules and Regulations law allowed NPs to prescribe.

TABLE 1.1 NP Pioneers

Nurse Practitioner Pioneers	Involvement
Loretta C. Ford, EdD, RN, PNP, FAAN, FAANP	American Academy of Nursing, the first pediatric nurse practitioner program
Deborah Kiley, DNP, NP-C, FNP-BC, FNAP, FAANP	American Academy of Nurse Practitioners
Judith Shannon Lynch, MS, MA, APRN-BC, FAAN	Board of Directors AANP, chair of the certification committee
Donna B. McArthur, PhD, FNP-BC, FNAP, FAANP	Vanderbilt University, ambulatory care center in the United States and Saudi Arabia
Richard (Rick) F. Meadows, MS, NP-C, FAANP	CEO of American Academy of Nurse Practitioners National Certification Board
Barbara Sheer, PhD, FNP, PNP, FAANP	President of the American Academy of Nurse Practitioners, Chair of the National Alliance of Nurse Practitioners, and international nurse practitioner

Many NP pioneers were educators. They were involved in the Academy of Nurse Practitioners either as leaders or members, pushing forward and setting the stage for practice as we know it today. All of these pioneers were active in creating and working within professional organizations working to reduce barriers and elevate the voices of NPs.

Nurse Practitioners

A "nurse practitioner" is a nurse with a graduate degree in advanced practice nursing, often referred to as an "advanced registered nurse practitioner" (ARNP) or "advanced practice registered nurse" (APRN). The American Association of Nurse Practitioners (AANP, 2019) reports that NPs provide healthcare services, including diagnosing and managing acute, chronic, and complex health problems; health promotion; disease prevention; health education; and counseling to individuals, families, groups, and communities. The American Association of Colleges of Nursing (AACN, 2022) envisions APNs advancing evidence-based solutions and leading innovation as we look to the future in the changing health care environment. Key goals include accelerating diversity and inclusion, transitioning to competency-based education and assessment, and increasing collaboration between education and practice (AACN, 2022).

History of Nursing Response to a Crisis

Nurses have a strong and distinguished history of stepping up in a crisis. In 1918, the great pandemic, better known as the "Spanish influenza pandemic of 1918–1919," spread worldwide and caused at least 50 million deaths worldwide, including 675,000 in the United States (Jones & Saines, 2019). Public health departments were unprepared for illnesses of this magnitude. World War I was underway, and medical personnel were in high demand. The Atlantic Red Cross, led by Lillian Ward of the Henry Street Settlement, mobilized nurses, volunteers, retired nurses who returned to work, and college students to help recruit more volunteers (Robinson, 1990). Nurses traveled to areas of need, transporting food supplies and providing care. The focus of nursing shifted to a patient-centered, rather than technically proficient, approach.

World War I increased the demand for nursing; approximately 23,000 nurses served. The war called for special skills, and nursing diversified to meet the need. As early as 1920, nurses delivered anesthesia, while nurse midwives delivered babies, and public health nursing expanded. Approximately 1,500 nurses died in World War I while caring for the sick and wounded. After World War II, new challenges required many nurses for increasingly complex and technical patient needs. Nursing was seen as a heroic profession and continued to flourish. Following Vietnam in the 1960s, highly trained combat medics developed into highly skilled physician assistants, and nurses began advanced practices that ultimately evolved into the position of NPs. Nurses learned to adapt and adjust to their surroundings, applying critical thinking and problem-solving skills and functioning closely with multidisciplinary team members (Ha & Nuntaboot, 2016). The roles and responsibilities of NPs and physician assistants have drastically evolved and are expected to continue to change in the face of current health care reform (Thorogood, 2014).

The recent pandemic follows the trends of the past. Many nurses and NPs were needed to provide patient care in response to patient demand and overloaded hospitals, particularly in rural areas. COVID-19, like Spanish influenza, has also claimed the lives of many health care workers. The World Health Organization (WHO, 2021) estimates that as many as 180,000 health and other care workers died from COVID-19 between January 2020 and May 2021.

The COVID-19 Pandemic: The Impact on Advanced Nursing Practice

In June 2022, the Department of Health and Human Services (DHHS) released a report, showing that over 3 million people enrolled in Affordable Care Act coverage and 21 million people enrolled in Medicaid Expansion coverage (DHHS, 2022). The influx of people with available insurance created an unprecedented primary care shortage.

On January 9, 2020, the WHO announced a mysterious corona-virus-related pneumonia in Wuhan, China. By January 21, 2020, the first virus cases had entered the United States on March 11, 2020, and the global pandemic became a public health emergency. Within 2 months, the number of COVID-19 cases had reached 100,000 and continued to climb. This dramatic increase in illness prompted a sudden growth in the need for health care services (Kleinpell et al., 2021; Poghosyan et al., 2021).

The COVID-19 pandemic highlighted significant vulnerabilities and disparities in our health care system. Differences within and between nations, rich and poor communities, and the healthy and seriously ill are growing (Rosa et al., 2020). COVID-19 had a devastating impact on health equity. Many people suffered social isolation and fear of illness and the loss of their insurance, homes, and jobs (Shadmi et al., 2020). Health care providers were in high demand, and recruitment efforts to travel to hot spots offered salaries of $5,000–$7,000 per week (Ackerman, 2021).

NP Practicc

Food for Thought

1. How can we address some of the disparities highlighted during COVID-19?
2. How do you think the end of the pandemic will affect NPs' scope of practice?

The WHO declared the novel coronavirus (COVID-19) a global health pandemic on March 11, 2020. The COVID-19 (SARS-CoV-2) pandemic dominated health care worldwide. The unprecedented global impact changed the face of health care, straining medical resources and prompting health care institutions to leverage workforce skills wherever possible (Rosa et al., 2020)—in the U.S., 17 states expanded the APRN scope of practice during the first 21 days of the pandemic (Feyereisen, 2020; Phillips, 2022; Rosa, 2020). The need for health care providers due to the COVID-19 pandemic created an environment in which emergency regulatory and policy changes expanded the NP scope of practice (Stucky et al., 2021). COVID-19 precipitated substantial changes. What happens next?

The APN/NP role came to fruition to increase access to health care for rural children and families. Nursing has a long and proud history of stepping up in a crisis, and NPs are uniquely qualified to fill the gap in our primary care system. NPs are the fastest-growing sector of primary care providers (AANP, 2021).

In the 2011 *The Future of Nursing* report by the Institute of Medicine, the message was, "Nurses should practice to the full extent of their education and training." (IOM, 2011, p. 4). The report stimulated many states' interest in granting full practice authority to NPs. Practice authority varies from state to state. There are three classifications of practice authority: full practice authority, reduced practice authority, and restricted practice authority:

- **full practice authority:** has no restrictions and allows NPs to evaluate, diagnose, order medication and diagnostic testing, and treat their patients. They fall under the oversight of their board of nursing or its equivalent (Kleinpell et al., 2021). There are 22 states and three territories that have full practice authority.
- **reduced practice authority:** requires NPs to collaborate or be under the supervision of a physician, creating a barrier. In 2020, there were 16 reduced practice states.

- **restricted practice:** states require strict collaboration or supervision of practice or limited practice. In 2020, there were 12 restricted practice states.

COVID-19 significantly burdens APNs, due to practice restrictions (Kleinpell et al., 2021; Poghosyan et al., 2022). The scope of practice restriction became a point of contention. In 2021, an executive order issued by governors of 21 reduced or restricted states removed or reduced the scope of practice restriction, allowing NPs to provide patient care.

Retired health care personnel were asked to return to work, and schools accelerated graduations. Several states relaxed regulations, removing physician supervision for NPs and

TABLE 1.2 Full Practice Authority

Alaska	Iowa	New Mexico
Arizona	Maine	North Dakota
Colorado	Maryland	Northern Mariana Islands
Connecticut	Massachusetts	Oregon
Delaware	Minnesota	Rhode Island
District of Columbia	Montana	South Dakota
Guam	Nebraska	Vermont
Hawaii	Nevada	Washington
Idaho	New Hampshire	Washington, DC
Kansas	New York	Wyoming
any federal facility, Veterans Administration medical center, Indian Health Service, etc.		

Note. Adapted from "AANP Policy Brief," https://storage.aanp.org/www/documents/advocacy/FPA-2022.pdf. "Nurse Practitioner Practice Authority: A State-by-State Guide," by Nurse Journal staff, https://nursejournal.org/nurse-practitioner/np-practice-authority-by-state/#:~:text=Currently%2C%20Alaska%2C%20Arizona%2C%20Colorado,D.C.%2C%20and%20Wyoming%20are%20full.

increasing prescribing privileges. Other states reduced the transition to practice hours required, and some reduced the supervision requirements. The order was intended to be a temporary fix but has provided the opportunity for NPs to collect data supporting independent practice.

TABLE 1.3 Reduced Practice Authority

Alabama	Louisiana	Utah
Arkansas (improved practice authority)	Mississippi	West Virginia
Illinois	New Jersey	Wisconsin
Indiana	Ohio	Virginia (improved practice authority)
Kentucky	Pennsylvania	

TABLE 1.4 Restricted Practice Authority

California	Missouri	Tennessee
Florida	North Carolina	Texas
Georgia	Oklahoma	Virginia
Michigan	South Carolina	

Massachusetts General Hospital's response to the pandemic involved creating and reassigning new roles for advanced practice providers (APP). APPs operated a COVID-19 hotline and staffed respiratory illness clinics (RICs). Additionally, they participated in results and care management and support teams, covered the isolation hotel, and performed vascular and enteric access procedures.

CRNA-Certified Registers Nurse Anesthetist

Certified registered nurse anesthetists (CRNAs) are advanced practice registered nurses, who work with various medical professionals, providing anesthesia for surgeries, special procedures, and dentistry. Approximately 59,000 CRNAs (CRNAs and CRNA students) work in practice. The nurse anesthetist role began in 1956, and in 1986, CRNAs became the first nursing specialty eligible for direct reimbursement from Medicare (ANA, 2023). At that time, the nurse anesthetist outnumbered the anesthesiologist; the numbers reversed by 2000. CRNAs face similar problems in recognition and scope of practice as other APRN designations.

CRNAs also work as members of interdisciplinary pain management teams for patients with chronic pain. CRNAs evaluate patients and provide pain treatment therapies, such as spinal injections with fluoroscopy (for imaging guidance), joint injections, and peripheral nerve blocks. Rural areas where providers are limited depend heavily on CRNAs to provide anesthesia service. CRNAs have full practice authority in all federal facilities but may still experience restricted practice based on state legislation. However, many CRNAs worked with an expanded scope of practice during the pandemic. CRNAs found themselves with expanded patient responsibilities during the COVID-19 pandemic.

Other Changes in Practice

Acute care NPs refocused their efforts on providing care for patients diagnosed with COVID. Education for the staff, families, and the general public became essential to preventing the spread of the disease. Early testing, surveillance, targeting, and quarantining of infected individuals took precedence (Diez-Sampedro et al., 2020). Nurses and NPs staffed testing and vaccine centers and provided supervision. Social distance and social isolation contributed to fear, dramatically decreasing the number of patients seen in primary care clinics.

Telepsychiatry and telehealth expanded and became a lifeline for therapeutic interventions and treatment (Diez-Sampedro et al., 2020). The impact of the pandemic on the health care workforce has been tremendous. Strained mental health and well-being of practitioners has been well documented, with anxiety, depression, mental exhaustion, work stress, fear of contamination, insomnia, burnout, and posttraumatic stress disorder being prevalent (Barrett & Heale, 2021; Diez-Sampedro et al., 2020; McGilton et al., 2021). New evidence-based practice protocols were developed and implemented (Diez-Sampedro et al., 2020). The devastating pandemic provided unprecedented opportunities for APN/NP innovation and change. The question is, where do we go from here?

Food for Thought

When the crisis emerged, granting APRN autonomy or reducing restrictions on practice became a moot point. This begs the question of why APRN practice was restricted in the first place.

INTERNATIONAL PRACTICE

The APN/NP role was developed to meet health care needs and continues to evolve. Its duties can range from providing care across the life span to specialty concentrations, such as treating the acutely ill or those suffering from chronic disease. The development of the NP role is progressing at various rates worldwide. In higher-income countries such as Canada, Australia, the United Kingdom, the Netherlands, and the United States, the NP is a registered nurse with graduate education, either at the master's or doctoral level. In 2020, the International Council of Nurses (ICN) published "Guidelines on Advanced Practice Nursing," indicating that the minimum requirement for entry into APN is a master's degree. This requirement is seen as aspirational in many low- and middle-income countries, due to a lack of funds (ICN, 2020). The NP role is evolving to fill gaps in the health care system and meet the needs of various populations.

The ICN Nurse Practitioner/Advanced Practice Network (ICN NP/APNN), launched in 2020, is an international resource for NPs that collaborates closely with the ICN. The titles of APNs vary worldwide, but the essential educational requirement is constant, with a minimum of a master's degree. The COVID-19 pandemic allowed practitioner to identify health disparities and gaps in existing health care systems, and countries needed help to leverage their resources to meet their needs.

Australia

The NP is a protected title in Australia in all states and territories in Australia and requires a master's level education. The NP role was discussed in 1990 and the first pilot project with 10 NP ran between 1992-1995. The NP role was initially designed to expand and increase access to health services, particularly for underserved populations (Currie, 2021). COVID-19 caused widespread disruptions to health services. The Australian College of Nurse Practitioners actively responded to the pandemic. During the initial phase of COVID-19, NP-led primary-care practices were denied personal protective equipment from the national stockpiles. Many NPs who practice in remote areas were restricted from crossing borders, which left some areas without health care. Rural regions are challenging, lack providers, limited access to care, low socioeconomic status and culture, create a demand for services that increased with the onset of COVID-19. An alternative and innovative NP-led model of care previously given little consideration was effective in providing service during the height of the pandemic. The Victoria Rural Health Service implemented an after-hours, NP-led model of care for its urgent care center (Wilson et al., 2021). Contracted NPs provided care on the weekends between 8 p.m. to 8 a.m., relieving some of the pressure on the existing health care system. Services provided included acute and aged care. The NPs' approach was considered holistic, evidence-based, and more current than the general practice counterparts (Wilson et al., 2021). COVID-19 has allowed the NPs to open a dialogue on the scope of practice and utilization of APNs.

Canada

In Canada, APNs encompass two roles, clinical nurse specialists (CNSs) and NPs, which began with outpost nursing over a century ago (Staples et al., 2020). The NP role may vary between provinces. Ontario has the greatest concentration of NPs and is the epicenter of NP regulation. The NPs in Canada have full autonomy to diagnose, treat, order, and interpret diagnostic tests and prescribe treatment and medication. However, there is a substantial variation in the scope of practice between Canadian provinces and territories. In 2020, there were 6,661 NPs licensed to practice in Canada (Murphy et al., 2022). Over half of licensed Canadian NPs reside in Ontario. In Quebec, Alberta, and British Columbia combined, there are approximately 1,828 NPs. Many NPs provide care to vulnerable and underserved populations but are still underutilized. Many NPs in Canada face similar issues related to the scope of practice as in the United States. Some provinces do not allow NPs to prescribe medication, order specific medical tests, or discharge patients from the hospital. Nursing groups are struggling to improve NPs' scope of practice and access to primary care.

The COVID-19 pandemic highlighted vulnerabilities and the ineffectiveness of the current Canadian health care system in addressing policies and the disproportionate impact on the health of underserved populations. The pandemic accentuated the problems in nursing workplace shortages and nursing education. During the pandemic, staffing shortages in all nursing roles created a recognition of the importance of global and regional strategies for strengthening our nursing workforce (Murphy et al., 2022). With an aging population, increasing chronic disease, and health disparities for indigenous people, NPs are critical in improving access to health care. There is a strong need to act, change the policies, and invest in nurses—particularly in increasing the RN and NP workforce—to prevent a health system collapse.

Excerpts from "Investing in Canada's Nursing Workforce Post-pandemic: A Call to Action"

"Invest in nurses—and in particular on increasing the RN and NP workforce—to prevent a health system collapse."

—Dr. Doris Grinspun

"This report demonstrates the urgent need for action to attract and retain nurses through investment and nursing leadership to ensure patient safety. Nurses must influence policy and key decisions in our health care system."

—Dr. Mélanie Lavoie-Tremblay

"If we in Canada want to return to our global reputation for excellence in health care, we need to cease treating nurses as commodities, embrace the abundance of literature showing the benefits of employing and supporting sufficient numbers of well-prepared nurses, and permit them to work to their full scope of practice."

—Dr. Judith Oulton

Note. From "Investing in Canada's Nursing Workforce Post-pandemic: A Call to Action," by Murphy et al., https://www.facetsjournal.com/doi/10.1139/facets-2022-0002.

China

The Ministry of Health of the People's Republic of China developed a strategic plan to produce 25,000 specialty nurses. The goal to "build a healthy China" and the struggle for identity between specialty nurses and APNs is slow to be recognized. The establishment of clinical master's programs in 2010 was a significant step in developing the NP role (Wong et al., 2018).

APNs in China have highly specialized knowledge and considerable responsibility for service development & delivery and professional development. A master's degree or above is required in health care policy, system leadership, and clinical scholarship (Mao, 2020; Wu, 2019; Wong et al., 2018).

The nursing roles in China are still developing and changing. Many health care workers were infected early in the pandemic, with the transmission route undetermined. Sichuan Provincial People's Hospital (SPPH) sent three teams to Wuhan as a COVID-19 emergency response led by nurse leaders and APNs. APNs are considered expert practitioners, consultants, managers, and leaders and have significantly contributed to public health. The nurse leaders and APNs evaluated and assigned staff based on competency levels. The teams triaged patients, established isolation wards, and adjusted shifts based on the severity of illness, establishing a very effective new workflow (Gao et al., 2020). *People's Daily*, a local paper, reported that APNs were invaluable and essential in managing and providing care for patients with COVID-19 (Mao, 2020).

The Netherlands

APNs in the Netherlands hold the title of certified nurse specialist (CNS), which is very similar to the NP role, requiring the completion of a 2-year dual master's program: the master advanced nursing practice (MANP). Upon completion, the APN specializes in their area of interest. APNs are required to register with a division of the Central Information Centre for Professional Practitioners. The role was introduced in 1997 due to the increasing number of chronically ill and aging patients (Van den Brink et al., 2019). It has been accepted and expanded, improving cost efficiency and outcomes (Maier, 2019; Van den Brink, 2019). The Dutch have incorporated the international experience into their leadership course to facilitate role development and leadership. In the last few decades, NPs have assumed the role of general practitioners to meet the rising demands for primary care (Teunissen, 2015). The scope of practice for Dutch NPs includes assessment and diagnosis, full prescriptive authority within their specialization (Maier, 2019), procedure and referrals, and autonomous practice without physician supervision (Van den Brink et al., 2019).

In response to the demands of the pandemic, Dutch NPs were instrumental in maintaining continuity of care despite the crisis and providing public health education as new information and best practices emerged. Nursing home deaths doubled during the first wave of the pandemic. The NPs working in long-term care environments worked diligently to control the spread of infection by developing and implementing emergency infection control strategies to manage the outbreak. NPs became a conduit for information, educating staff and the community. They stepped up to fill gaps in health care, encouraging virtual collaboration with their physician counterparts and emotional support for staff and families (McGilton et al., 2021).

Republic of Ireland

In 1998, the Commission of Nursing recommended that the registered advanced NP role be developed. The first post was in minor emergency care. Since then, the role has continued growing. The Nurse and Midwifery Board of Ireland published the National Standard and requirements for identifying a master-level education for RANP practice (ICN 2020), which is in keeping with the recommendations of the International Council of Nurses. The educational foundation is competency based, focusing on (a) autonomy in clinical practice within a collaboratively agreed scope of practice; (b) expert practice, which provides both practical and theoretical expertise on nursing practice and the role of advanced nursing practice; (c) professional and clinical leadership, which provides leadership and management skills appropriate to seek out and improve patient care and management in new and innovative ways; and (d) research, which provides a level of expertise to implement evidence-based practices within the workplace (ICN, 2020; INAP, 2022).

During the pandemic, the Irish health care system was recovering from underfunding and experiencing significant capacity constraints (Humphries et al., 2021). At their conference, the TD Minister for Health, Stephen Donnelly, addressed the Irish Nurses and Midwives Organisation (INMO) to praise them for their work during COVID-19. The INMO worked diligently coordinating, planning, and rolling out the vaccination program (the Irish vaccine program was highly effective in fighting COVID-19, and Ireland has one of the lowest rates of infection globally). Donnelly (2022) indicated that health service reform is vital and focuses on increasing hiring, adding more hospital beds, and developing a safe staffing framework. Nurses and midwives play an essential role in developing the framework, including in the context of enhanced, specialist, and advanced practice. Donnelly (2022) requested an increase in the number of advanced nurse and midwifery practitioners in the workforce, from 2% to 3%, and provided funding to add around 160 additional advanced nursing and midwifery practitioners (Donnelly, 2022).

The United Kingdom: England, Scotland, Wales, and Northern Ireland

In the United Kingdom, the role of the NP was established in the early 1990s and is less developed than in the United States (Lawler et al., 2020). There needs to be more standardization in education and practice, which leads to role confusion. Health Education England (HEE) developed a national framework for advanced clinical practice in 2017, which it defines as

> a level of practice characterized by a high degree of autonomy and complex decision making. This is

> underpinned by a master's level award or equivalent that encompasses the four pillars of clinical practice, leadership, and management, education, and research, demonstrating core capabilities and area-specific clinical competence. (HEE, 2017)

The role of advanced clinical practitioners includes nurses and other health professionals struggling with their identity.

NPs working with the frail elderly adapted. The change was swift and decisive. Within three months, the practitioners established a new service that included video consultations and were able to spend more time with patients in need. They also implemented an infection control prevention and screening system to ensure patient and staff safety and a new triaging system to streamline and prioritize patients' access to acute services (Morley et al., 2022). Additionally, they proposed a research objective to examine patients' responses to the virtual nurse-led clinic (Wood et al., 2021).

As with many APNs, innovation, flexibility, and adaptability became the key to providing care. Concerns over the lack of personal protective equipment and the mental health of nurses and providers continue to be an issue as the severity of the pandemic diminishes.

TABLE 1.5 Country Comparison

Country	Formal Education	Title	No of APNs	Nationally certified	Regulation	Additional
United States	Master's or doctorate level	Advanced practice registered nurse/nurse practitioner nurse anesthetist nurse midwife clinical nurse specialist	355,000 NPs licensed in the United States	National certification	Federal and State level jurisdiction	
Australia	Master's level	Nurse practitioner	2,250+ NPs endorsed in Australia.	National certification	Federal and Jurisdictional	

(Continued)

TABLE 1.5 Country Comparison (*Continued*)

Country	Formal Education	Title	No of APNs	Nationally certified	Regulation	Additional
Canada	Master's level	Nurse practitioner clinical nurse specialist	7,400 NPs	National certification	Federal and Province level jurisdictional	
China	Master's level	Nurse specialist	50,000 RNs have completed APN training	Unknown	unknown	
Ireland	Master's level	Registered advanced nurse practitioners	1700 RANPs	National certification		
United Kingdom	Master's level	advanced practice nurses Nurse specialists Advanced practice physiotherapists	There is no separate registry outside of that of the general nursing registry.	No	No	Multidisciplinary advanced practice framework

CHAPTER SUMMARY

Dubbed the "International Year of the Nurse and the Midwife," 2020 brought with it enormous challenges caused by the onset of the COVID-19 (SARS-CoV-2) pandemic. NPs stepped up to meet the challenge in the United States and worldwide. The role of the NP continues to evolve, and circumstances that led to the initial development of the role in the 60s are being replicated today. An aging population and chronic disease prevalence increase the need for primary care providers. COVID-19 has dramatically affected the health care system and clearly illustrated the presence of health disparities and lack of access to care for many racial, ethnic, and marginal groups. The U.S. Department of Labor expects NP positions to increase by 52% by 2030 (BLS, 2022).

In many countries, NPs function autonomously to increase access to health care. In several lower-income countries, there is an increased interest in developing APN roles to improve access to care. Still, resources are limited.

The COVID-19 pandemic and the increasing complexity of global issues illustrate that collaborative solutions are essential to education and health care as we advance in the 21st century (WHO, 2019). The importance of international cooperation and collaboration is intuitive and widely supported (Bump et al., 2021). Wilson and colleagues (2020) report, "Nurses are caring science professionals, and they are a valuable contribution to world health, representing the largest disciplinary proportion (59%) of the health professions sector." A adequate strategy for creating an adequate health care workforce is ensure the right health workers are in the right places and to expand the roles of health workers to meet patient needs (Anonymous, 2022).

KEY POINTS

- Historically, the NP's role has evolved in response to changing health care needs.
- Physician shortages, health disparities, and unmet needs drive health care change.
- Organizations provide support and help facilitate change.
- Globally, NPs face the same challenges and tackle problems through innovation and collaboration.

ACTIVITIES

1. Reflect on the impact COVID-19 has had on the role of the NP. Should the changes to the position be permanent? How would you encourage and support their permanency?
2. Choose a country not mentioned in the chapter and review the development of the NP role and the educational requirements. Be prepared to discuss the differences in education and practice.

REFERENCES

Ackerman, T. (2021). Job offers of up to $12,000 a week lure Houston nurses to COVID-19 hot spots. *Houston Chronicle*. https://www.houstonchronicle.com/news/houston-texas/health/article/Job-offers-of-up-to-12-000-a-week-lure-Houston-15875348.php

American Association of Colleges of Nursing. (2022). *AACNs vision for academic nursing*. https://www.aacnnursing.org/News-Information/Position-Statements-White-Papers/Vision-for-Nursing-Education

The American Association of Nurse Practitioners. (2019). *Scope of practice for nurse practitioners accessed*. https://www.aanp.org/advocacy/advocacy-resource/position-statements/scope-of-practice-for-nurse-practitioners#:~:text=Professional%20Role&text=NPs%20provide%20a%20wide%20range,%2C%20families%2C%20groups%20and%20communities

Anonymous. (2022). NP positioning for the future health care workforce. *The Nurse Practitioner*, *47* (1), 4. https://doi.org/10.1097/01.NPR.0000803004.16833.0d

Barrett, D. (2021). The role of health care leaders and managers during COVID-19. *University of Hull Online Blog*. https://online.hull.ac.uk/blog/the-role-of-health care-leaders-and-managers-during-covid-19

Barrett, D., & Heale, R. (2021). COVID-19: Reflections on its impact on nursing. *Evidence-based Nursing*, *24*(4), 112–113. https://doi.org/10.1136/ebnurs-2021-10346

Berg, J. A. (2020). The perils of not knowing the history of the nurse practitioner role. *Journal of the American Association of Nurse Practitioners*, *32*(9), 602–609. https://doi.org/10.1097/JXX.0000000000000004

Bernhardt, J. M., Chittle, M., Marden, J., & Sawicki, D. (2020). COVID-19 pandemic creates new roles for advanced practice providers. *Clinical Advisor*. https://www.clinicaladvisor.com/home/topics/infectious-diseases-information-center/roles-advanced-practice-providers-covid-19-pandemic/

Bureau of Labor Statistics, U.S. Department of Labor. *Occupational Outlook Handbook. Nurse Anesthetists, Nurse Midwives, and Nurse Practitioners*. www.bls.gov/ooh/fastest-growing.html

Currie, J. (2021). Patients' access to care during COVID-19 and the role of nurse practitioners in Australia. *Journal of Law and Medicine, 28*(2), 336–345.

Dalen, J. E., Ryan, K. J., & Alpert, J. S. (2017). Where have the generalists gone? They became specialists, then subspecialists. *The American Journal of Medicine, 130*(7), 766–768. https://doi.org/10.1016/j.amjmed.2017.01.026

Department of Health and Human Services. (2022). *New reports show record 35 million people enrolled in coverage related to the affordable care act, with historic 21 million people enrolled in Medicaid expansion coverage.* https://www.hhs.gov/about/news/2022/04/29/new-reports-show-record-35-million-people-enrolled-in-coverage-related-to-the-affordable-care-act.html#:~:text=media%40hhs.gov-,New%20Reports%20Show%20Record%2035%20Million%20People%20Enrolled%20in%20Coverage,Enrolled%20in%20Medicaid%20Expansion%20Coverage

Donnelly, S. (2022). *Statement from the minister of health to IMNOs annual delegate conference.* https://www.gov.ie/en/speech/530e1-statement-from-minister-for-health-to-inmos-annual-delegate-conference/

Edmonds, M. (2015). Nurse practitioner pioneers—Celebrating 50 years of role development. *The Journal for Nurse Practitioners, 11*(6), 578–595. https://doi.org/10.1016/j.nurpra.2015.04.004

Ford, L. (1979). A nurse for all settings: The nurse practitioner. *Nursing Outlook*, 27, 516–521.

Feyereisen, S., & Puro, N. (2020). Seventeen states enacted executive orders expanding advanced practice nurses' scopes of practice during the first 21 days of the COVID-19 pandemic. *Rural and Remote Health, 20*, 6068. https://doi.org/10.22605/RRH6068

Gao, X., Jiang, L., Hu, Y., Li, L., & Hou, L. (2020). Nurses' experiences regarding shift patterns in isolation wards during the COVID-19 pandemic in China: A qualitative study. *Journal of Clinical Nursing, 29*(21–22), 4270–4280. https://doi.org/10.1111/jocn.15464

Ha, D., & Nuntaboot, K. (2016). How nurses in hospital in Vietnam learn to improve their own nursing competency: An ethnographic study. *Journal of Nursing & Care, 5*(5) https://doi.org/10.4172/2167-1168.1000368

Health Education England. (2017). Multi-professional framework for advanced clinical practice in England. https://www.hee.nhs.uk/sites/default/files/documents/multi-professionalframeworkforadvancedclinicalpracticeinengland.pdf

Jones, M. M., & Saines, M. (2019). The eighteen of 1918–1919: Black nurses and the great flu pandemic in the United States. *American Journal of Public Health, 109*(6), 877–884. https://doi.org/10.2105/AJPH.2019.305003

Kleinpell, R., Myers, C. R., Schorn, M. N., & Likes, W. (2021). Impact of COVID-19 pandemic on APRN practice: Results from a national survey. *Nursing Outlook, 69*(5), 783–792. https://doi.org/10.1016/j.outlook.2021.05.002

Hoffman B. (2003). Health care reform and social movements in the United States. *American Journal of Public Health, 93*(1), 75–85. https://doi.org/10.2105/ajph.93.1.75

Humphries, N., Creese, J., Byrne, J. P., & Connell, J. (2021). COVID-19 and doctor emigration: the case of Ireland. *Human Resources for Health, 19*(1), 29. https://doi.org/10.1186/s12960-021-00573-4

International Advance Practice Nursing. (2020). Advanced practice nursing in the Netherlands. https://internationalapn.org/2022/07/01/netherlands/

International Advanced Practice Nursing. (2022). Advanced practice nursing in Ireland. https://internationalapn.org/2014/06/29/ireland/

International Council of Nurses. (2020). Guidelines on advanced practice nursing. https://www.icn.ch/system/files/documents/2020-04/ICN_APN%20Report_EN_WEB.pdf

Lawler, J., Maclaine, K., & Leary, A. (2020). Workforce experience of the implementation of an advanced clinical practice framework in England: A mixed methods evaluation. *Human Resources for Health, 18*(1), 96. https://doi.org/10.1186/s12960-020-00539-y

Lopes-Júnior L. C. (2021). Advanced practice nursing and the expansion of the role of nurses in primary health care in the Americas. *SAGE Open Nursing, 7*, 23779608211019491. https://doi.org/10.1177/23779608211019491

Maier C. B. (2019). Nurse prescribing of medicines in 13 European countries. *Human Resources for Health, 17*(1), 95. https://doi.org/10.1186/s12960-019-0429-6

Mannix, R., Lee, L. K., & Fleegler, E. W. (2020). COVID-19 and firearms in the United States: Will an epidemic of suicide follow? *Annals of Internal Medicine, 173*(3), 228–229. https://doi.org/10.7326/M20-1678

Mao, X., Yang, Q., Li, X., Chen, X., Guo, C., Wen, X., & Loke, A. Y. (2021). An illumination of the ICN's core competencies in disaster nursing version 2.0: Advanced nursing response to COVID-19 outbreak in China. *Journal of Nursing Management, 29*(3), 412–420. https://doi.org/10.1111/jonm.13195

McGilton, K. S., Krassikova, A., Boscart, V., Sidani, S., Iaboni, A., Vellani, S., & Escrig-Pinol, A. (2021). Nurse practitioners rising to the challenge during the Coronavirus Disease 2019 pandemic in long-term care homes. *The Gerontologist, 61*(4), 615–623. https://doi.org/10.1093/geront/gnab030

McKnight-Eily, L. R., Okoro, C. A., Strine, T. W., Verlenden, J., Hollis, N. D., Njai, R., Mitchell, E. W., Board, A., Puddy, R., & Thomas, C. (2021). Racial and ethnic disparities in the prevalence of stress and worry, mental health conditions, and increased substance use among adults during the COVID-19 pandemic: United States, April and May 2020. *MMWR. Morbidity and Mortality Weekly Report, 70*(5), 162–166. https://doi.org/10.15585/mmwr.mm7005a3

Morley, D. A., Kilgore, C., Edwards, M., Collins, P., Scammell, J. M., Fletcher, K., & Board, M. (2022). The changing role of Advanced Clinical Practitioners working with older people during the COVID- 19 pandemic: A qualitative research study. *International Journal of Nursing Studies, 130*, 104235. https://doi.org/10.1016/j.ijnurstu.2022.104235

Murphy, G. T., Sampallib, T., Bearskinc, L. B., Cashen, N., Cummings, G., Rose, A. E., Etowag, J., Grinspunh, D., Jones, E. W., Lavoie-Tremblay, M., MacMillan, K., MacQuarrle, C., Martin-Misener, R., Oulton, J., Ricciardellio, R., Silasp, L., Thorne, S., & Villeneuve, M. (2022). Investing in Canada's nursing workforce post-pandemic: A call to action. *Facets, 7, 1051–1120.* https://doi.org/10.1139/facets-2022-0002

Peck, J. L., & Sonney, J. (2021). Exhausted and burned out: COVID-19 emerging impacts threaten the health of the pediatric advanced practice registered nursing workforce. *Journal of Pediatric Health Care: Official Publication of National Association of Pediatric Nurse Associates & Practitioners, 35*(4), 414–424. https://doi.org/10.1016/j.pedhc.2021.04.012

Phillips S. J. (2022). 34th Annual APRN Legislative Update: Trends in APRN practice authority during the COVID-19 global pandemic. *The Nurse Practitioner, 47*(1), 21–47. https://doi.org/10.1097/01.NPR.0000802996.14636.1c

Poghosyan, L., Pulcini, J., Chan, G. K., Dunphy, L., Martsolf, G. R., Greco, K., Todd, B. A., Brown, S. C., Fitzgerald, M., McMenamin, A. L., & Solari-Twadell, P. A. (2022). State responses to COVID-19: Potential benefits of continuing full practice authority for primary care nurse practitioners. *Nursing Outlook, 70*(1), 28–35. https://doi.org/10.1016/j.outlook.2021.07.012

Raine, S., Liu, A., Mintz, J., Wahood, W., Huntley, K., & Haffizulla, F. (2020). Racial and Ethnic Disparities in COVID-19 Outcomes: Social Determination of Health. *International Journal of Environmental Research and Public Health, 17*(21), 8115. https://doi.org/10.3390/ijerph17218115

Stevens R. A. (1996). Health care in the early 1960s. *Health Care Financing Review, 18*(2), 11–22.

Ter Maten, A., & Garcia-Maas, L. (2009). Dutch advanced nursing practice students: Role development through international short-term immersion. *The Journal of Nursing Education, 48*(4), 226–231. https://doi.org/10.3928/01484834-20090401-11

Rosa, W. E., Fitzgerald, M., Davis, S., Farley, J. E., Khanyola, J., Kwong, J., Moreland, P. J., Rogers, M., Sibanda, B., & Turale, S. (2020). Leveraging nurse practitioner capacities to achieve global health for all: COVID-19 and beyond. *International Nursing Review, 67*(4), 554–559. https://doi.org/10.1111/inr.12632

Teunissen, D. T., Stegeman, M. M., Bor, H. H., Toine, & A. L. M., Lagro-Janssen. (2015). Treatment by a nurse practitioner in primary care improves the severity and impact of urinary incontinence in women. An observational study. *BMC Urology, 15*, 51. https://doi.org/10.1186/s12894-015-0047-0

Van den Brink, G. T. W. J., Kouwen, A. J., Hooker, R. S., Vermeulen, H. & Laurant, M.G.H. (2019). An activity analysis of Dutch hospital-based physician assistants and nurse practitioners. *Human Resources for Health*. 78(2019). https://doi.org/10.1186/s12960-019-0423-z

World Health Organization. (2021). The impact of COVID-19 on health and care workers: A closer look at deaths. https://apps.who.int/iris/handle/10665/345300

Wilson, E., Hanson, L. C., Tori, K. E., & Perrin, B. M. (2021). Nurse practitioner led model of after-hours emergency care in an Australian rural urgent care centre: Health service stakeholder perceptions. *BMC Health Services Research*, *21*(1), 819. https://doi.org/10.1186/s12913-021-06864-9

Wong, F. (2018). Development of advanced nursing practice in China: Act local and think global. *International Journal of Nursing Sciences*, *5*(2), 101–104. https://doi.org/10.1016/j.ijnss.2018.03.003

Woo, B., Poon, S. N., Tam, W., & Zhou, W. (2021). The impact of COVID-19 on advanced practice nursing education and practice: A qualitative study. *International Nursing Review*. Advance online publication. https://doi.org/10.1111/inr.12732

Wood, E., King, R., Senek, M., Robertson, S., Taylor, B., Tod, A., & Ryan, A. (2021). UK advanced practice nurses' experiences of the COVID-19 pandemic: a mixed-methods cross-sectional study. *BMJ Open*, *11*(3), e044139. https://doi.org/10.1136/bmjopen-2020-044139

Wang, H., English, M., Chakma, S., Namedre, M., Hill, E., & Nagraj, S. (2022). The roles of physician associates and advanced nurse practitioners in the National Health Service in the UK: A scoping review and narrative synthesis. *Human Resources for Health*, *20*(1), 69. https://doi.org/10.1186/s12960-022-00766-5

Yang, B. K., Johantgen, M. E., Trinkoff, A. M., Idzik, S. R., Wince, J., & Tomlinson, C. (2021). State nurse practitioner practice regulations and U.S. health care delivery outcomes: A systematic review. *Medical Care Research and Review: MCRR*, *78*(3), 183–196. https://doi.org/10.1177/1077558719901216

CHAPTER 2

Advanced Practice Nursing Education Pathway

MSN and BSN to DNP

Carole Mackavey and Linda Cole

OBJECTIVES

Upon completion of the chapter, the student will be able to

1. discuss the rationale behind the move to DNP as an entry-level degree
2. discuss the impact of the DNP on nursing leadership
3. review the NP/Advanced Nursing Practice Certification and specialty
4. understand the impact of the pandemic on the advanced practice education path

QUESTIONS/CHALLENGES

1. What are your thoughts on the BSN to DNP as the new entry level for advanced practice nursing?
2. What is the best way to engage students in an online learning environment?
3. How do you think the pandemic influenced nursing education?
4. What changes would you make to the current degree structure, and why?

INTRODUCTION

Advanced practice nursing education programs prepare nurses to function beyond entry-level professional nursing practice (American Association of Colleges of Nursing [AACN], 2021, p. 21). The programs prepare graduates for training in an advanced nursing specialty, such as administration/practice leadership, informatics, or an advanced practice nursing role: certified nurse practitioner, certified nurse-midwife, certified clinical nurse specialist, or certified registered nurse anesthetist (AACN, 2021, pp. 21–22).

There has been a long-standing debate surrounding entry-level degrees for APNs. There has been resistance to the change, citing retiring faculty and the faculty shortage as significant barriers. Many smaller universities think the doctor of nursing practice (DNP), as an entry-level degree, will significantly impact their financial structure. The deadline for transitioning from entry-level APN to DNP is 2025, but this is not the first time a deadline has been proposed. There has been some progress toward the desired outcome, and the new BSN-to-DNP program is emerging. There is a consensus between the American Association of Colleges of Nursing (AACN) and the National Organization of Nurse Practitioner Faculty (NONPF) regarding the desired outcomes for nursing education. They have revised the essentials in response to communities feeling that nurses and advanced practice nurses need to prepare for entry to practice in today's medical environment. The new *Essentials: Core Competencies for Professional Nursing Education* reflects the need for competency-based education. (See Chapter 3 for additional information on competency-based education.) Whether accomplishing this goal by 2025 is possible and its impacts on smaller colleges and universities is still to be determined.

THE MOVE TOWARD DOCTORAL EDUCATION

Today's health care environment requires APNs and other practitioners to function with the highest education, knowledge, and practice expertise to provide quality patient outcomes (AACN, 2022). The DNP degree path was in conception for some time. In 2005, the National Academy of Sciences recommended that nursing education develop a non-research clinical doctorate (AACN, 2022). The Doctor of Nursing Practice (DNP) is a terminal degree emphasizing clinical expertise and leadership skills. The DNP degree follows the path of other health professions that transitioned to doctoral degrees, such as physical therapy (DPT), pharmacy (PharmD), and psychology (PsyD) (Edwards, 2018). Psy DNP is a practice doctorate.

In 2018, the NONPF presented the shift to the DNP by 2025 to entry-level nurse practitioner (NP) programs. The DNP degree can be obtained in one of two ways: via a direct path (BSN to DNP) or stages (the BSN to MSN followed by an MSN to DNP). While variation in DNP roles has led to variations across DNP curricula, there are two main foci of this degree: (a) advance practice registered nurses (APRN), nurse practitioners, clinical nurse specialists, nurse midwives, and nurse anesthetists and (b) executive leadership (preparing chief nursing officers and other top-level managers (Edwards et al., 2018). The DNP prepares students to be practice leaders, create innovative patient care models, develop cost-effective ways to manage patients through quality improvement and impact health policy. The move to DNP supports the Institute of Medicine (IOM) mandate for nursing's unique perspective to be added to the interprofessional approach, thus improving the nation's health (IOM, 2010).

The transition to the DNP as entry level has been slow, and many are there must be more financial incentives for the advanced degree (Nelson, 2023). There has been some question about whether the DNP-prepared APN practitioner improves the quality of care (Nelson, 2023). The DNP degree focuses on clinical expertise and leadership skills. DNP programs prepare APNs to translate evidence into practice as leaders for patient care teams, evaluate patient outcomes, and promote quality and safety along with system change (Fasching, 2022).

Boswell et al. (2020) conducted focus groups to review the impact of the DNP degree on health care in West Texas. The DNP systems thinking approach to care delivery resulted in decreased errors, improved interdisciplinary communication and collaboration, and improved patient outcomes. The DNP-prepared APN demonstrated strong leadership skills through innovation and coordinated decision-making skills.

The need for leadership across organizations and health care systems was evident during the recent pandemic. New roles and positions were created, and new models of care were developed. APNs worked to fill the gap by working with communities to meet the complex, rapidly evolving health care environment. The DNP-prepared APN provides systems-level thinking, financial planning, management, and organizational skills.

CHALLENGES FACED BY THE DNP

Even though the DNP degree was developed based on an early IOM report, the *Future of Nursing Report, 2010* didn't mention the practice doctorate (McCaughey et al., 2020). The inconsistencies in the degree have created barriers, the move forward has been prolonged, and many universities maintained their master's in nursing program despite instituting a DNP program. Discrepancies in education and the variety and various types of DNP projects have led to uncertainty in the health care community. A clear definition and purpose of the DNP-prepared graduate has been a struggle. DNP graduates work in a diverse number of positions and continue to develop new positions and pathways. Some states' limitations in the scope of practice have inhibited growth and acceptance.

CLINICAL ROLE OF THE ADVANCED PRACTICE NURSE/NP

Increasing access to primary health care continues to be a serious concern. The recent focus on advanced practice nursing is on preparing the APN to meet the demanding needs of today's health care system. The recent pandemic highlighted many existing health disparities and identified increasing issues directly related to the pandemic. The increase in homelessness, health care access inequities, domestic violence, hunger, and racism dramatically rose with the pandemic. Advanced practice nurses very often provide care for underserved populations and rural health.

APN roles vary worldwide, using different titles to identify the role. The most common titles are nurse practitioner (NP), advanced practice nurse (APN), advanced practice registered nurse (APRN), and clinical nurse specialist (CNS; ICN, 2020). Advanced practice registered nurses and nurse practitioners are similar, but different professions and are often used interchangeably.

NPs are a type of APRN/APN. However, NPs generally are primary caregivers and work in hospitals, primary care offices, and health care clinics. There are different specialties under the NP umbrella. Each specialization has a national certification examination, and the role and responsibilities can vary based on that certification. All advanced practice nurses will need continuing education and must be recertified every 5 years.

TABLE 2.1 Nurse Practitioner Specialty Certification

family nurse practitioner (FNP)
adult gerontology nurse practitioner (AGNP)
adult gerontology acute care nurse practitioner (AGNP)
emergency nurse practitioner (ENP)
Psychiatricmental health nurse practitioner (PMHNP)
pediatric nurse practitioner (PNP)
neonatal nurse practitioner (NNP)

Advanced practice registered nurse/advanced practice nurses have four primary specializations. APRNs may work in hospitals but can also work as primary health care providers.

TABLE 2.2 Four Primary Specializations APN/APRN

nurse practitioners (NP)
certified nurse midwives (CNM)
clinical nurse specialists (CNS)
certified registered nurse anesthetists (CRNA)

NP SPECIALTY ADVANCED PRACTICE ROLES

Over time, there have been additions to the typical NP role with the health care system changes.

Nurse Educators

The education of health care providers, including nurses and advanced practice nurses, is constantly evolving (World Health Organization [WHO], 2016). Nurse educators hold an advanced degree, either a master's or doctorate, and are charged with inspiring, teaching, and mentoring others.

The World Health Organization (WHO) developed Nurse Educator Core Competencies. The competencies are designed for the preparation of nurse educators and were developed and validated using the Delphi method.

Nurse Educator Core Competencies

- **domain 1:** theories and principles of adult learning
- **domain 2:** curriculum design and implementation
- **domain 3:** nursing practice
- **domain 4:** research and evidence
- **domain 5:** communication, collaboration, and partnership

- **domain 6:** ethical/legal principles and professionalism
- **domain 7:** monitoring and evaluation
- **domain 8:** management, leadership, and advocacy

Nurse educators are responsible for keeping up with the constantly changing healthcare expectations, demographics, technological advancements, practice requirements, and rapidly growing amount of evidence-based information (Leong et al., 2021; WHO, 2016).

The new AACN *Essentials*, outlining the move to competency-based education, is transforming nursing education. There is a strong argument for teaching clinical and diagnostic reasoning to prepare the student better to meet the needs of the health care system.

The impacts of COVID-19 forced nursing educators to move the course content from a face-to-face or hybrid model to an online venue. The rapid change has created considerable challenges for students and faculty. Some challenges included finding a place at home to work or study; obtaining a reliable internet connection; and a need for more structure, creating problems for some and encouraging others. Synchronous versus asynchronous lectures, student engagement, virtual simulation, and other forms of active learning are critically important.

NP Nurse Executive Leadership

As health care continues to evolve, the demand for nurse leaders has increased. Nurse executive doctors of nursing practice (DNP) are uniquely positioned to effect change. The program prepares students for executive leadership and decision-making by examining practice innovations and outcomes. The DNP leadership degree focuses on organizational culture, innovation, systems thinking, ethics, collaboration with a multi-disciplinary team, and other administrative skills (Shelby & Wermer, 2020). Nurse executives (NE) serve on hospital boards and use their expertise for quality improvement, patient safety, health care administration and policy, and management (Foxx & Gardner, 2021). Many of the courses are online, but clinical experience in leadership is vital to competency. (See Chapter 7 for more on the role of the APN in leadership.) NE also serves on the community advisory board, leads nursing organizations, and advocates for much-needed change. The impact of DNP-prepared leaders can reach state, regional, national, and global areas (Boswell et al., 2021).

During the recent pandemic, nurse leaders redesigned care delivery to meet the care needs of patients. They prioritized patient needs and developed new roles to manage staffing shortages and overwhelming workloads. (For more information on nursing leadership, see Chapter 7.)

NP Nursing Informatics

The rapid changes in information technology and the need for quick access to scientific knowledge have created a demand for experts who can bridge the gap between clinical and technology. EHRs were adopted in 2004 and further advanced in 2009. The role of nurses in informatics continues to grow and evolve. Nurses' clinical experience allows them to identify gaps in health care information. Data is becoming increasingly helpful in health care improvement.

The American Nurses Association (ANA) defines "nursing informatics" as "the specialty that integrates nursing science with multiple information and analytical sciences to identify, define, manage and communicate data, information, knowledge, and wisdom in nursing practice" (2002). Nurse informatics has two levels: undergraduate and graduate. The graduate level is an informatics nurse specialist or nurse informaticist, bringing medical knowledge to information technology experience and a master's or doctorate (American Nurses Association [ANA], 2021). The role of the nurse informaticist is growing and expanding. Menkiena (2021) identified three key responsibilities: communicate the "why" associated with new processes, help with the implementation, and assess data quality. There is also a competency-based Informatics Nursing Board Certification examination.

Certified Nurse–Midwives (CNM) and Women's Health Nurse Practitioners

Certified nurse–midwives provide primary health care for women from teens through young adulthood and menopause; care during pregnancy, including birth and the postpartum period; care of the newborn during the first 28 days of life; gynecology and family planning services; and treatment of male partners for sexually transmitted infections (Marzalik et al., 2018). The CNM requires an advanced degree from a midwifery program and passing the required certification exams. There are currently only 40 educational programs in the United States.

Women Health Nurse Practitioners (WHNP)

Women's Health Nurse Practitioners (WHNP) are trained and specialize in women's health care and assess, diagnose, and treat the health care needs of women across the lifespan. They provide primary care services and specialize in obstetrics, gynecology, and care for episodic or chronic illnesses.

Clinical Nurse Specialists (CNS)

Clinical nurse specialists (CNSs) require an advanced nursing degree, typically a master's or doctoral degree and must pass a certification examination. The role can be traced back to the 1930s, with role definition and educational requirements established in the late 1960s (Cooper et al., 2019; Mohr & Coke, 2018). They have similar training to NPs and can diagnose, treat, and prescribe medication to patients. The scope of the CNS role ranges from wellness to illness and acute to chronic care (National Association of Clinical Nurse Specialists [NACNS], 2019). The CNS role focuses on three spheres of impact: direct patient care, organizations and systems, and nurses and nursing practice (NACNS, 2019). The CNS is educated in at least one of six population foci described in the APRN Consensus Model and then becomes certified by examination based on the population, which includes adult/gerontology, pediatric, or neonatal (NACNS, 2019). The APRN Consensus Model states that clinical nurse specialists who practice in most states must obtain certification based on population. Recertification is done every 5 years and includes requirements for continuing education hours (up to 150 hours, including 25 hours in pharmacotherapeutics) and practice hours (American Association of Critical Care Nurses [AACCN], 2023; American Nurses Credentialing Center [ANCC], 2022). CNS may obtain advanced clinical expertise with specialty certification in a focused area of nursing practice, such as pain management or palliative care, like any registered nurse pursuing specialty certification.

While there are similarities between CNSs and NPs, the CNS integrates care across the continuum through the continuous improvement in patient outcomes and nursing care by impacting the three spheres of impact (Mohr & Coke, 2018). These three spheres of impact (patient–client, nurses–nursing practice, and organizational–systems) define the scope and outcomes of the CNS. The patient–client sphere refers to providing direct clinical care. In the nurses–nursing practice sphere, the CNS works directly with bedside staff to improve care standards and provide education and support to nursing staff. Through the organizational–systems sphere, the CNS influences decisions at the organizational level, thus removing barriers to care, enhancing quality initiatives, and improving outcomes for patient populations. The CNS demonstrates impact at the microsystem (unit-level), mesosystem (organizational integration), and macrosystem (across systems, populations, or communities) levels of health care delivery (Mohr & Coke, 2018).

As with other APRNs, the COVID-19 pandemic impacted the CNS in various ways. In some cases, the CNS shifted into the role of bedside clinicians to provide direct patient care (Bruwer & Yates, 2020). Innovative care delivery strategies were also created, such as early identification of patients with clinical manifestations of COVID-19 through patient rounds and COVID-19 code blue teams (Mamais et al., 2022). Others moved into a support role for the bedside nurse, assisting wherever needed and role modeling positive behaviors and authentic leadership (Ladak et al., 2021). At the organizational level, CNSs were involved in protocol development for personal protective equipment preservation and implementation of best practices for infection prevention. They were deployed into administrative and supervisory roles (Bruwer & Yates, 2020).

Certified Registered Nurse Anesthetists (CRNA)

CNRAs are some of the primary anesthesia providers within the United States, particularly in rural areas. Certified Registered Nurse Anesthetists specialize in providing anesthesia to patients with trauma or undergoing surgery. In the United States, the CRNA entry level is a doctorate in nursing practice. The fundamentals of the CRNA program are slightly different than those of the NP. Students take the three Ps (pathophysiology, pharmacology, physical exam, and health assessment), but the focus is on the anesthesia.

The student registered nurse anesthetist (SRNA) needs 7–8½ years of coursework and clinical hours—on average, 9,400 hours. Other practice requirements include the following (AANA, 2023):

- a baccalaureate or graduate degree in nursing or another appropriate major

- an unencumbered license as a registered professional nurse and/or APRN in the United States or its territories
- at least one year of full-time work experience (or its part-time equivalent) as a registered nurse in a critical care setting
- graduation with a minimum of a master's degree from a nurse anesthesia educational program accredited by the Council on Accreditation of Nurse Anesthesia Educational Programs (COA)

The move toward a DNP is designed to align advanced practice nurses with other medical providers, such as physical therapists and pharmacists, requiring a doctorate. The doctorally prepared NP has the knowledge and skills needed to navigate the changing health care system and provide leadership into the future.

RECENT PANDEMICS' IMPACT ON NP EDUCATION

Lockdowns, mandatory mask-wearing, travel bans, and social distancing rapidly changed higher education (Woo, 2021). On-campus activities suddenly ceased or moved to an online format. Faculty struggled to transfer courses to the virtual environment, and the challenge of engaging students in an online environment became paramount when eliminating face-to-face campus-based teaching. Adjusting to the new climate presents questions, and faculty struggles to maintain quality in an often-unfamiliar platform. Students embraced the transition to online learning. Some students loved the flexibility, while others missed the human interaction.

A qualitative study by Woo et al. (2021) explored nursing student perceptions of COVID-19 impact in Singapore. Three major themes were identified, and each had two subthemes: overcoming adversity through innovation, accepting remote learning, and the versatility of APN practice in an ongoing pandemic. These findings were consistent with the University of California, Davis 2020 study that reviewed connectedness, effectiveness, and engagement in online learning.

CHAPTER SUMMARY

The impact of the pandemic was global. Most colleges and universities moved to online learning; however, the pace at which the university could change varied from country to country, depending on the available resources and technology (Sanders & Patel, 2020). Moving to online education requires considerable commitment and some experience with online education. Developing content for students that is engaging and thought provoking is challenging. Shared experiences help facilitate the success of online learning. When we think of graduate education during the pandemic, we invariably refer to online learning. What impact did COVID-19 have on the students themselves? Social isolation is difficult for some and almost impossible for others. Fear, stress, anxiety, and depression were common amongst students (Enujioke et al., 2021). Many APNs worked the front lines during the pandemic, and the preparedness to practice was challenged, requiring significant coping with staffing and equipment shortages and possible quarantine. COVID-19 provided many unique opportunities—innovations that might otherwise have taken years to emerge.

Food for Thought

1. What were the positive and negative effects of the COVID-19 pandemic on education?
2. What was your greatest challenge, and how did you overcome it?

KEY POINTS

- The concept of competency-based learning always starts with clearly defining the learning outcomes.
- Competency-based learning helps learners prepare for real-world interaction.
- Much of the assessment should be formative and provide an opportunity for remediation.

ACTIVITIES

1. Describe the type of education interaction that would stimulate learning in the online environment.
2. Do you prefer online learning or face to face and why?

REFERENCES

American Association of Colleges of Nursing [AACN]. (2021). *The essentials: Core competencies for professional nursing education.* https://www.aacnnursing.org/Portals/42/AcademicNursing/pdf/Essentials-2021.pdf

American Association of Colleges of Nursing [AACN]. (2022). Facts sheet: The doctor of nursing practice (DNP). https://www.aacnnursing.org/Portals/42/News/Factsheets/DNP-Fact-Sheet.pdf

American Association of Critical Care Nurses [AACCN]. (2023). *Acute/critical care clinical nurses specialist renewal handbook.* https://www.aacn.org/certification/certification-renewal/ccns-adult?tab=Practice%20Hours%20%26%20CE%20Points

American Nurses Association [ANA]. (2002). Nursing informatics: Scope and standards of practice (2nd ed.). https://www.nursingworld.org/nurses-books/nursing-informatics-scope-and-standards-of-practice-2nd-ed/

American Nurse Credentialing Center [ANCC]. (2022). Adult-gerontology clinical nurse specialist certification renewal requirements. https://www.nursingworld.org/our-certifications/adult-gerontology-clinical-nurse-specialist/

Bekemeier, B., Kuehnert, P., Zahner, S. J., Johnson, K. H., Kaneshiro, J., & Swider, S. M. (2021). A critical gap: Advanced practice nurses focused on the public's health. *Nursing Outlook, 69*(5), 865–874. https://doi.org/10.1016/j.outlook.2021.03.023

Boswell, C., Mintz-Binder, R., Batcheller, J., Allen, P., & Baker, K. A. (2021). Capturing the impact of the doctor of nursing practice degree on West Texas health care. *Journal of Continuing Education in Nursing, 52*(4), 192–197. https://doi.org/10.3928/00220124-20210315-08

Bove, L. (2020). Integration of informatics content in baccalaureate and graduate nursing education. *Nurse Educator, 45*(4), 206–209. https://doi.org/10.1097/NNE.0000000000000734

Bruwer, L., & Yates, E. (2020). Versatility of the clinical nurse specialist: It takes a pandemic. *Clinical Nurse Specialist, 34*(6), 244–245. https://doi.org/10.1097/NUR.0000000000000562

Cooper, M. A., McDowell, J., Raeside, L., & ANP-CNS Group. (2019). The similarities and differences between advanced nurse practitioners and clinical nurse specialists. *British Journal of Nursing, 28*(20), 1308–1314.

Edwards, N. E., Coddington, J. A., Erler, C. J., & Kirkpatrick, J. M. (2018). The impact of the role of doctor of nursing practice nurses on health care and leadership. *Medical Research Archives, 6*.

Enujioke, S. C., McBrayer, K., Soe, K. C., Imburgia, T. M., & Robbins, C. (2021). Impact of COVID-19 on postgraduate medical education and training. *BMC Medical Education, 21*(1), 580. https://doi.org/10.1186/s12909-021-03019-6

Fasching, F. (2022) DNP by 2025? 4 reasons to support DNP entry-to-practice nurse practitioner online. https://www.nursepractitioneronline.com/articles/4-reasons-to-support-dnp/

Foxx, M., & Garner, C. (2021). Qualifications of executive nurses for service on hospital boards. *The Journal of Nursing Administration, 51*(12), 626–629. https://doi.org/10.1097/NNA.0000000000001085

Hughes, R., Meadows, M. T., & Begley, R. (2022). AONL nurse leader competencies: Core competencies for nurse leadership. *Nurse Leader, 20*(5), 437–443. https://doi.org/10.1016/j.mnl.2022.08.005

Institute of Medicine [IOM]. (2010). *The future of nursing: Leading change, advancing health.* National Academies Press.

Kannampallil, T. G., Goss, C. W., Evanoff, B. A., Strickland, J. R., McAlister, R. P., & Duncan, J. (2020). Exposure to COVID-19 patients increases physician trainee stress and burnout. *PloS One*, *15*(8), e0237301. https://doi.org/10.1371/journal.pone.0237301

Kupferschmid, B., Creech, C., Lesley, M., Filter, M., & Aplin-Kalisz, C. (2017). Evaluation of doctor of nursing practice students' competencies in an online informatics course. *The Journal of Nursing Education*, *56*(6), 364–367. https://doi.org/10.3928/01484834-20170518-09

Ladak, A., Lee, B., & Sasinski, J. (2021). Clinical nurse specialists expands to crisis management role during COVID-19 pandemic. *Clinical Nurse Specialist*, *35*(6), 291–299. https://doi.org/10.1097/NUR.0000000000000632

Mamais, F., Jasdhaul, M., Gawlinski, A., Lawanson-Nichols, M., Kao, Y., Branom, R., & Ansryan, L. Z. (2022). The agile clinical nurse specialist: Navigating the challenges of the COVID-19 pandemic. *Clinical Nurse Specialist*, *36*(4), 190–195. https://doi.org/10.1097/NUR.0000000000000682

Menkiena, C. (2021). The three essential responsibilities of a nurse informaticist. *Health Catalyst*. https://www.healthcatalyst.com/insights/nurse-informaticist-3-essential-responsibilities#the-evolution-nurse-informaticist

Mohr, L. D., & Coke, L. A. (2018). Distinguishing the clinical nurse specialist from other graduate nursing roles. *Clinical Nurse Specialist*, *32*(3), 139–151. https://doi.org/10.1097/NUR.0000000000000373

Nelson, R. (2023). Doctorate for nurse practitioners slowly advances as entry-level degree. *Medscape Medical News*. https://www.medscape.com/viewarticle/986546?icd=login_success_email_match_norm

Nelson, T., & Parker, C. (2019). Nursing informatics: The EHR and beyond. *American Nurse*. https://www.myamericannurse.com/wp-content/uploads/2019/03/ant3-Informatics-Career-211.pdf

Pordeli, L. (2018). Informatics competency-based assessment: Evaluations and determination of nursing informatics competency gaps among practicing nurse informaticists. *Online Journal of Nursing Informatics*, *22*(3), 5.

Sandars, J., & Patel, R. (2020). The challenge of online learning for medical education during the COVID-19 pandemic. *International Journal of Medical Education*, *11*, 169–170. https://doi.org/10.5116/ijme.5f20.55f2

Shelby, M., & Wermers, R. (2020). Complexity science fosters professional advanced nurse practitioner role emergence. *Nursing Administration Quarterly*, *44*(2), 149–158. https://doi.org/10.1097/NAQ.0000000000000413

Shillam, C. R., & MacLean, L. (2018). Leadership influence: A core foundation for advocacy. *Nursing Administration Quarterly*, *42*(2), 150–153. https://doi.org/10.1097/NAQ.0000000000000276

Staggers, N., & Thompson, C. B. (2002). The evolution of definitions for nursing informatics: A critical analysis and revised definition. *Journal of the American Medical Informatics Association*, *9*(3), 255–261. https://doi.org/10.1197/jamia.m0946

Udod, S., MacPhee, M., & Baxter, P. (2021). Rethinking resilience. *JONA: Journal of Nursing Administration*, *51*(11), 537–540. https://doi.org/10.1097/NNA.0000000000001060

CHAPTER 3

AACN Competencies in Advanced Practice Nursing Education and Role

Carole Mackavey

OBJECTIVES

Upon completion of the chapter, the student will be able to

1. analyze challenges in assessing competencies in the classroom
2. analyze the challenges of evaluating competencies in the clinical setting
3. discuss the importance of the new AACN essentials and domains
4. integrate an understanding of clinical reasoning in advancing nursing's influence competency in health care

QUESTIONS/CHALLENGES

1. Why is competency education important to your role development?
2. Why is competency education essential to the practice and the public?

INTRODUCTION

Nurse practitioner (NP) graduates are trained to develop the knowledge, skills, and attitudes essential to autonomous clinical practice. Competency is achieved by developing critical thinking, clinical reasoning, and diagnostics reasoning skills. Critical thinking is a complex process, and the foundation of problem-solving that incorporates inquiry, analysis, and interpretation of data and information and applies that knowledge to solving a specific problem or situation. It is through the use of critical thinking skills that clinical reasoning and judgment are formed. Working with clinical preceptors, NP students can apply the knowledge acquired through mentored patient care experiences (Raterink, 2016).

COMPETENCY IN EDUCATION AND PRACTICE

Every NP program aims to produce high-quality clinicians prepared to practice in the constantly changing, complex, and fast-paced health care environment (D'Aoust et al., 2021). Competency requires strong communication skills, creative thinking, and clinical reasoning. Mastering these skills requires the practitioner to understand key concepts and apply the knowledge to significant clinical problems.

WHAT IS COMPETENCY-BASED EDUCATION (CBE)

Interest in competency-based education has been growing in the United States and internationally. Competency-based education definitions have been disputed, but the most widely accepted definition came from medicine. Frank et al. (2010) defined competency-based education (CBE) as an approach to preparing clinicians for practice, oriented toward graduate outcome abilities and organized around competencies derived from analyzing societal and patient needs. It de-emphasizes time-based training and promises greater accountability, flexibility, and learner-centeredness (Frank et al., 2010).

Competency in education means focusing on the students' learning and mastery of the content instead of focusing on grades. One of the main principles of competency-based education is that each student receives what they need to succeed to meet the desired outcome. The focus of education must be on measurable goals and outcomes. In genuine competency-based education, students move through the program at their own pace until competency is met. Competency assumes the student has completed a minimum performance based on predetermined standards established based on the needs of a population, region, national or international (Timmerberg et al., 2022).

Why Competency?

There is considerable variety in advanced practice nursing programs, and the move to competency will help define the advanced practice nurse role, strengthen their professional identity, and elevate practice readiness (American Nurses Association [ANA], n.d.). Students focus on clearly delineated learning and performance expectations for education and practice (AACN, 2021).

The American Association of Colleges of Nursing (2021) developed ten domains of competence:

- **domain 1:** knowledge for nursing practice
- **domain 2:** person-centered care
- **domain 3:** population health
- **domain 4:** scholarship for nursing discipline
- **domain 5:** quality and safety
- **domain 6:** interprofessional partnerships
- **domain 7:** systems-based practice

- **domain 8:** informatics and health care technologies
- **domain 9:** professionalism
- **domain 10:** personal, professional, and leadership development

The National Organization of Nurse Practitioner Faculty (NONPF) expanded and realigned its essentials to support the AACN. The table below outlines NONPF and AACN domains and competencies. Within the domains, there are competencies and subcompetencies. The first subcompetency is undergraduate nursing education, and the second is the graduate level, which explicitly targets the DNP graduate level. Each domain of competence has descriptors that define the domain. Each of the domains contain several competencies; for example, knowledge of nursing includes the following student competency: "Demonstrate an understanding of the discipline of nursing and the NP's role in distinct perspectives and where shared views exist with other disciplines." This competency then contains the following subcompetencies:

- Integrate historical, foundational, and population-focused knowledge into NP practice.
- Translate evidence from nursing science and other sciences into NP practice.
- Evaluate the application of nursing science to NP practice.

NONPF's Nurse Practitioner Role, Core Competencies Table is presented with the AACN Essentials level 2 subcompetencies in the left column and the NP role competencies in the right column. This design shows how the NP Role Core Competencies are scaffolded from the AACN Essentials.

NP Programs are to meet all the Essential competencies as well as to NONPF's NP Role Core Competencies

	AACN Essentials Advanced-Level Nursing Education	NONPF Nurse Practitioner (NP) Role Core Competencies
Domain 1	Domain 1: Knowledge for Nursing Practice Descriptor: Integration, translation, and application of established and evolving disciplinary nursing knowledge and ways of knowing, as well as knowledge from other disciplines, including a foundation in liberal arts and natural and social sciences. This distinguishes the practice of professional nursing and forms the basis for clinical judgment and innovation in nursing practice.	NP Domain 1: Knowledge of Practice The nurse practitioner integrates, translates, and applies established and evolving scientific knowledge from diverse sources as the basis for ethical clinical judgement, innovation, and diagnostic reasoning.
	1.1 Demonstrate an understanding of the discipline of nursing's distinct perspective and where shared perspectives exist with other disciplines	NP 1.1 Demonstrate an understanding of the discipline of nursing's and the NP's role distinct perspective and where shared perspectives exist with other disciplines
	1.1e Translate evidence from nursing science as well as other sciences into practice.	NP 1.1h: Integrate historical, foundational and population focused knowledge into NP practice.
	1.1f Demonstrate the application of nursing science to practice.	NP 1.1i: Translate evidence from nursing science and other sciences into NP practice.

National Organization of Nurse Practitioner Faculties, Selection from "NONPF Nurse Practitioner Role Core Competencies Table."

(*Continued*)

NP Programs are to meet all the Essential competencies as well as to NONPF's NP Role Core Competencies (*Continued*)

	AACN Essentials Advanced-Level Nursing Education	NONPF Nurse Practitioner (NP) Role Core Competencies
Domain 1	1.1g Integrate an understanding of nursing history in advancing nursing's influence in health care.	NP 1.1j: Evaluate the application of nursing science to NP practice.
	1.2 Apply theory and research-based knowledge from nursing, the arts, humanities, and other sciences.	NP 1.2 Apply theory and research-based knowledge from nursing, the arts, humanities, and other sciences.
	1.2f Synthesize knowledge from nursing and other disciplines to inform education, practice, and research.	NP 1.2k: Synthesize evidence from nursing and other disciplines to inform and improve NP practice at a micro, meso, and macro level.
	1.2g Apply a systematic and defendable approach to nursing practice decisions.	NP 1.2l: Translate science-based theories and concepts to guide one's overall NP practice.
	1.2h Employ ethical decision making to assess, intervene, and evaluate nursing care.	NP 1.2m: Employ ethical decision making to manage and evaluate patient care and population health.
	1.2i Demonstrate socially responsible leadership.	NP 1.2n: Practice socially responsible leadership.
	1.2j Translate theories from nursing and other disciplines to practice.	

American Association of Colleges of Nursing, "Selection," The Essentials: Core Competencies for Professional Nursing Education, pp. 27. Copyright © 2021 by American Association of Colleges of Nursing (AACN). Reprinted with permission.

Competency-Based Clinical Education

Competency is a student-centered, gradual, step-by-step process in which students are expected to apply academic knowledge to clinical situations. The student's clinical experience is influenced by their previous experience as a nurse and their preceptors. New NP students will likely experience the "imposter phenomenon," while moving from the role of an experienced nurse to a new NP student. The imposter phenomenon is a psychological experience that occurs when "high-achieving individuals doubt their skills, talents, or abilities and fear being exposed as a fraud" (Peregrin, 2022). Students usually develop clinical competency when providing direct patient care. Their preceptors provide support and confidence; competency is gained and progresses gradually during each subsequent clinical rotation. One of the challenges in developing clinical competency is the increase in the incidence of chronic disease and the advancing age of the population.

Previous clinical education has been passive and time-oriented, resulting in various acquired skills. The errors in skills and procedures put patient safety at risk. The World Health Organization discussed the importance of simulation techniques to achieve mastery of skills without risk to patients (WHO, 2009). Students would have to demonstrate mastery of skills with the goal of all students meeting the clearly defined set of outcomes. Mastery or competency has no time limit and is focused on outcomes, limiting skill variability (Friederichs, 2018).

In competency-based education, faculty and learners form a partnership in which the faculty provides structure and support to facilitate their progression toward unsupervised practice. Clinical scenarios, simulations, and preceptors all play an essential role in the learner's development. "Clinical reasoning" is the foundation of clinical competency, the decision-making process requiring mental reasoning. A range of approaches are used in clinical reasoning. The dual process theory is the most widely recognized approach and involves two thinking approaches. System 1 thinking is fast, requires little mental effort, is intuitive, and entails an emotional response to situations and stimuli. System 1 is linked to pattern recognition, while system 2 is analytically slow, requires effort, and focuses on cause and effect (Congdon et al., 2022; Norman et al., 2017; ten Cate, 2017; Thampy et al., 2019). Frequently, in the practice of experienced providers, system 1 thinking prevails, unless system 1 fails to meet the mark, at which point system 2 will be implemented. With the system, one encounters the possibility of biases, such as cognitive biases, which can lead to diagnostic errors.

An example of a cognitive bias is confirmation bias, wherein information is interpreted to fit a preconceived diagnosis, causing a practitioner to order tests to support the initial diagnosis. Another is anchoring bias, which refers to the tendency to make decisions based on this information or the search for evidence to confirm the early diagnosis (Thampy et al., 2019). Cognitive bias is a challenge to system 1 thinking. Everyone has biases, and they can affect the decision-making process. Practitioners and learners need to be aware of their biases; the key is incorporating both systems of thinking in the diagnostic because clinical reasoning is both a process and an outcome (ten Cate & During, 2017, p. 35). Clinical reasoning requires a strong foundation of knowledge from core courses, such as pathophysiology, physical examination, and pharmacology.

CHAPTER SUMMARY

The re-envisioned AACN competencies, *The Essentials: Core Competencies for Professional Nursing Education*, has stimulated higher education to look at how learners are prepared for the challenge of today's health care environment. The competencies apply to all areas of nursing and advanced practice nursing, providing the programs with a guide to developing a competent provider.

Food for Thought

1. What are some of the ways competency can be confirmed?
2. How do you demonstrate all that you have learned?

KEY POINTS

- The concept of competency-based learning always starts with clearly defining the learning outcomes.
- Competency-based learning helps learners prepare for real-world interaction.
- Much of the assessment should be formative and provide an opportunity for remediation.

ACTIVITIES

1. Create reflection questions relating to your learning stage based on what you have learned in this chapter.
2. Consider how does the competency framework affects your learning process.
3. Does the competency framework support entry-level practice?

REFERENCES

Chaney, K. P., & Hodgson, J. L. (2021). Using the five core components of competency-based medical education to support implementation of CBVE. *Frontiers in Veterinary Science*, *8*, 689356. https://doi.org/10.3389/fvets.2021.689356

D'Aoust, R. F., Brown, K. M., McIltrot, K., Adamji, J. D., Johnson, H., Seibert, D. C., & Ling, C. G. (2022). A competency roadmap for advanced practice nursing education using PRIME-NP. *Nursing Outlook, 70*(2), 337–346. https://doi.org/10.1016/j.outlook.2021.10.009

Groenewegen, A. (2022). Kahneman fast and slow thinking explained. *Sue Behavioural Design* https://suebehaviouraldesign.com/kahneman-fast-slow-thinking/

Hall, A., Rich, J., Dagnone, J., Weersink, K., Caudle, J., Sherbino, J., Frank, J., Bandiera, G., & Van Melle, E. (2020). It's a marathon, not a sprint: rapid evaluation of competency-based medical education program implementation. *Academic Medicine, 95*(5), 786–793. https://doi.org/10.1097/ACM.0000000000003040

Hauer, K. E., Lockspeiser, T. M., & Chen, H. C. (2021). The COVID-19 pandemic as an imperative to advance medical student assessment: Three areas for change. *Academic Medicine: Journal of the Association of American Medical Colleges, 96*(2), 182–185. https://doi.org/10.1097/ACM.0000000000003764

Holmboe, E. S. (2021). The transformational path ahead: Competency-based medical education in family medicine. *Family Medicine, 53*(7), 583–589. https://doi.org/10.22454/FamMed.2021.296914

Kavanagh, J. M., & Szweda, C. (2017). A crisis in competency: The strategic and ethical imperative to assessing new graduate nurses' clinical reasoning. *Nursing Education Perspectives, 38*(2), 57–62. https://doi.org/10.1097/01.NEP.0000000000000112

Olson, A., Rencic, J., Cosby, K., Rusz, D., Papa, F., Croskerry, P., Zierler, B., Harkless, G., Giuliano, M., Schoenbaum, S., Colford, C., Cahill, M., Gerstner, L., Grice, G., & Graber, M. (2019). Competencies for improving diagnosis: an interprofessional framework for education and training in health care. *Diagnosis, 6*(4), 335–341. https://doi.org/10.1515/dx-2018-0107

Raterink, G. (2016). Reflective journaling for critical thinking development in advanced practice registered nurse students. *Journal of Nursing Education., 55*(2), 101–4. https://doi.org/10.3928/01484834-20160114-08. PMID: 26814821.

Ryan, M. S., Holmboe, E. S., & Chandra, S. (2022). Competency-based medical education: Considering its past, present, and a post-COVID-19 era. *Academic Medicine: Journal of the Association of American Medical Colleges, 97*(3S), S90–S97. https://doi.org/10.1097/ACM.0000000000004535

Singh, H., Meyer, A. N., & Thomas, E. J. (2014). The frequency of diagnostic errors in outpatient care: Estimations from three large observational studies involving U.S.

adult populations. *BMJ Quality & Safety, 23*(9), 727–731. https://doi.org/10.1136/bmjqs-2013-002627

ten Cate, O. (2017). Competency-based postgraduate medical education: Past, present and future. *GMS Journal for Medical Education, 34*(5), Doc69. https://doi.org/10.3205/zma001146

ten Cate, O. (2017). Introduction. In O. ten Cate et al. (Eds.), *Principles and practice of case-based clinical reasoning education: A method for preclinical students* (pp. 3–19). Springer.

ten Cate, O., & Durning, S. J. (2017). Understanding clinical reasoning from multiple perspectives: A conceptual and theoretical overview. In O. ten Cate et al. (Eds.), *Principles and practice of case-based clinical reasoning education: A method for preclinical students* (pp. 35–46). Springer.

Timmerberg, J. F., Chesbro, S. B., Jensen, G. M., Dole, R. L., & Jette, D. U. (2022). Competency-based education and practice in physical therapy: It's time to act! *Physical Therapy, 102*(5), pzac018. https://doi.org/10.1093/ptj/pzac018

Thampy, H., Willert, E., & Ramani, S. (2019). Assessing clinical reasoning: Targeting the higher levels of the pyramid. *Journal of General Internal Medicine, 34*(8), 1631–1636. https://doi.org/10.1007/s11606-019-04953-4

van Melle, E., Frank, J. R., Holmboe, E. S., Dagnone, D., Stockley, D., Sherbino, J., & International Competency-Based Medical Education Collaborators. (2019). A core components framework for evaluating implementation of competency-based medical education programs. *Academic Medicine: Journal of the Association of American Medical Colleges, 94*(7), 1002–1009. https://doi.org/10.1097/ACM.0000000000002743

Woo, B. F. Y., Lee, J. X. Y., & Tam, W. W. S. (2017). The impact of the advanced practice nursing role on quality of care, clinical outcomes, patient satisfaction, and cost in the emergency and critical care settings: A systematic review. *Human Resource Health, 15*(1), 63. https://doi.org/10.1186/s12960-017-0237-9. PMID: 28893270; PMCID: PMC5594520.

Yazdani, S., & Hoseini Abardeh, M. (2019). Five decades of research and theorization on clinical reasoning: A critical review. *Advances in Medical Education and Practice, 10*, 703–716. https://doi.org/10.2147/AMEP.S213492. PMID: 31695548; PMCID: PMC6717718.

CHAPTER 4

Simulation in Advanced Practice Nursing

Mandi Lyons and Padma Ramaswamy

OBJECTIVES

Upon completion of the chapter, the student will be able to

1. define the term "simulation"
2. discuss the evolution of simulation in health care and nursing
3. describe the critical role of simulation in education and practice
4. discuss the process of developing patient simulations
5. describe reflective practice in simulation
6. discuss the growth in simulation post-COVID-19 pandemic

Food for Thought

1. What does the word "simulation" mean to you?
2. How has simulation shaped health care education as it is today?

QUESTIONS/CHALLENGES

1. Think of a patient encounter you have had during your career that has made an impact on your professional development. What did you learn from that situation? As you move throughout the chapter, begin to think how simulation-based education can be used to recreate that experience for others to learn from.

INTRODUCTION

Simulation is a sophisticated pedagogical teaching methodology that creates artificial experiences that represent real-life scenarios for learning. During simulation, the learner engages in expertly guided learning activities reflecting real-world experiences but without the consequences of an actual situation. Simulation-based learning in nursing has become a valuable technique in preparing nurses to provide care within a complex health care system. The literature has several definitions based on the various aspects of simulation. Gaba (2007), associate dean for immersive and simulation-based learning at Standford Medicine, defines simulation as "a technique, not a technology, to replace or amplify real experiences with guided experiences, often immersive in nature, that evoke or replicate substantial aspects of the real world in a fully interactive fashion" (p. 126). Lioce et al. (2020) define simulation as "a technique that creates a situation or environment to allow persons to experience a representation of a real event for practice, learning, evaluation, testing, or to gain an understanding of systems or human actions "(p. 44). The International Nursing Association for Clinical Simulation and Learning (INASCL, 2016) defines simulation as "a pedagogy using one or more typologies to promote, improve, or validate a participant's progression from novice to expert." Regardless of how it is defined, the purpose of simulation in health care is to provide a safe environment that creates standardized experiences for all learners to enhance their knowledge, teamwork, technical and nontechnical skills to optimize patient safety and quality care (Gaba, 2007; Lioce et al., 2020).

Simulation has been slowly adopted for nursing; however, since 2010, its use as a teaching pedagogy has caused it to evolve and become a new standard in the education and training of undergraduate and graduate nursing students (Sanko, 2017). However, research regarding the effectiveness of simulation-based education (SBE) on advanced practice nursing (APN) educational outcomes, transition to practice, and essential nursing competencies is limited. Therefore, the utilization of simulation in APN education is not widespread and sporadic (Lioce et al., 2020; National Task Force on Quality Nurse Practitioner Education [NTF], 2016). This chapter focuses on the current state of simulation in APN programs and the potential for simulation integration into educational and practice settings to enhance nursing and patient outcomes. Furthermore, this chapter provides an overview of simulation modalities and methodology as well as a peek into the future of simulation growth.

HISTORICAL FOUNDATIONS OF SIMULATION

Many industries have used simulation to prepare individuals for their future jobs, where critical errors could result in catastrophic events. Aviation, military, nuclear power industry, and the U.S. space programs utilize simulation to polish team training, performance safety, and crisis management. Moreover, simulation creates a safe environment to conduct "what if" scenarios that could be too costly or dangerous to perform in a real-world setting (Aebersold, 2016; Herrera-Aliaga & Estrada, 2022; Nickerson & Pollard, 2010; Sanko, 2017). These industries share one important similarity with health care: people's lives depend on quick decision-making, skill aptitude, and hasty reaction time to life-threatening situations (Nickerson & Pollard, 2010).

Simulation is integral in improving patient safety through team training. One of the notable contributions to simulation is the National Aeronautics and Space Administration's (NASA) Cockpit Resource Management principles, which have been adopted by health care to benefit intensive care, surgical, and anesthesia teams (Table 4.1; Ayaz & Ismail, 2022).

TABLE 4.1 Crew Resource Management Principles Utilized in Health Care

Concept	Definition	Expectation	Rationale
Communication	Bottom up and top down Assertiveness; transparent	Active listening—repetition of the sender's message back to them for understanding	Ensures information is communicated regardless of position in team; raises situation awareness
Leadership	Ensure all team members are used optimally and heard	Organizing appropriate tasks for team members, supportive manner, functioning	Provide monitors and mentors, trust, develop self and team assessment to obtain maximum results
Briefing	Maintain a common plan; rebrief with new conditions	Knows personal role/ other's roles as well as the expectations of roles, teams, and outcomes.	Times when to pause and rebrief when conditions or goals change. Reduce Potential errors/ threats to avoid

(Continued)

TABLE 4.1 **Crew Resource Management Principles Utilized in Health Care (*Continued*)**

Concept	Definition	Expectation	Rationale
Mutual Monitoring	Observations of self and others; call out errors (errors are expected)	Give and receive advice in an open, nonjudgmental manner	Aims to prevent potential errors and threats as well as engage in backup behaviors
Team Adaptability	Workload/tasks shift based on conditions and workload capacities	Monitoring and knowing when to shift and assist to achieve a desired goal	Redistributes workloads and continuously re-evaluates to adapt
Decision-Making	Collecting and utilizing all information within its current state	Bringing up relevant information and alternative actions	Makes the best decision possible for the best outcome; considers "what is right" not "who is right"
Debriefing	Continuous process improvement	Reflection of actions/outcomes	Reforms and reorganizes for optimal outcomes

Adapted from Harris, D. (2018). Crew Resource Management for Automated Teammates (CRMA). In (Vol. 10906, pp. 215–229). Switzerland: Springer International Publishing AG.

EVOLUTION OF SIMULATION IN NURSING

Simulation as a teaching method has been used in nursing for over a century. One of the earliest reports of simulation use is of a midwife named Madam du Courdray, who used a pelvic "machine" to train midwives on safer birthing practices during the 18th century throughout France (Maxworthy et al., 2023). Beginning in the 19th century, the "mother of nursing," Florence

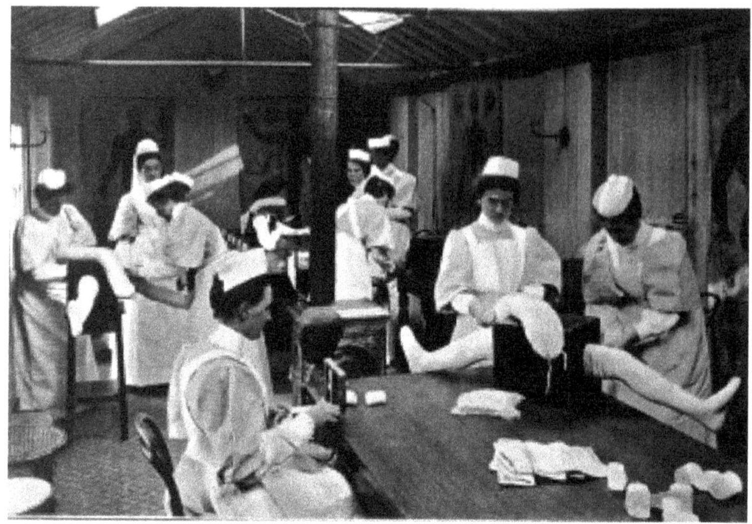

FIGURE 4.1 A bandaging class with leg models at the London Hospital Nurse Training program.

Nightengale, advocated for training nurses to use "jointed skeletons" and limb models to practice bandaging, bathing, and mobility needs (Figure 4.1; Herrera-Algia & Estrada, 2022; Maxworthy et al., 2023; Sanko, 2017).

After a century of using straw-filled models, Connecticut's Hartford Hospital nurse training program commissioned a doll-maker named Martha Jenkins Chase to create a life-sized manikin, known as Ms. Chase, made of a hard plastic. Ms. Chase was designed to mimic the adult human form with mobile joints that allowed student nurses to practice fundamental skills, such as dressing and undressing, transporting, and turning patients (Herrera-Aliaga & Estrada, 2022; Nickerson & Pollard, 2010; Sanko, 2017; Singleton, 2020). By the 1920s and 1930s, adult-size and infant manikins (Figure 4.2) could be found throughout hospital training schools. Similar to simulation labs of today, dedicated spaces, known as "demonstration rooms," were created to store practice equipment, manikins, and allow nurses to observe and practice fundamental skills (Nickerson & Pollard, 2010; Singleton, 2020).

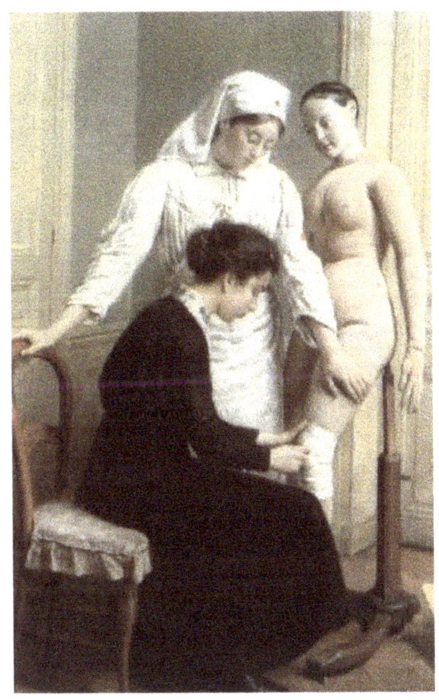

FIGURE 4.2 Adult manikin used to demonstrate skills.

With the increased demand for competent, experienced nurses after World War II, nursing training programs relied heavily on demonstrations, manikins, and task trainers to train nurses to deal with complex health problems (Singleton, 2020). The Hill-Burton Act (aka the Hospital Survey and Construction Act of 1946) provided construction grants and loans to build more hospitals, nursing homes, and other health facilities, increasing the need for trained nurses (Health Resources and Services Administration [HRSA], 2022). This increase in hospitals and health care facilities led to further demand for nursing training programs. However, the rise of medical errors and preventable deaths steadily increased.

After the landmark report *To Err is Human: Building a Safer Health System* was published in 1999, the focus shifted toward using simulation in nursing programs to help prevent medical errors within the health care system (Sanko, 2017). The increased use of simulation received the attention of nursing leaders to collaborate and develop standards of best practices for SBE in nursing. Figure 4.3 depicts the timeline of historic nursing and simulation events.

By 2002, the International Nursing Association of Clinical Simulation and Learning (INASCL), which continuously regulates the standards for nursing simulation, was formed (Sanko, 2017). The increasing demand for simulation prompted companies, such as Laerdal™ and Medical Education Technologies, Inc. (METI),

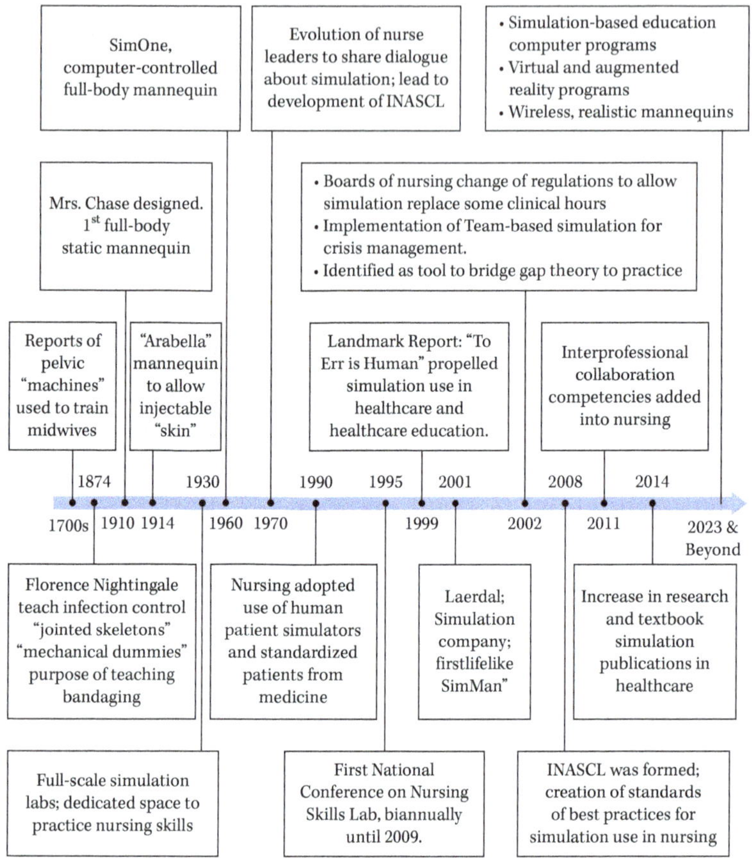

FIGURE 4.3 Timeline of historic nursing and simulation events (Herrera-Aliaga & Estrada, 2022; Nickerson & Pollard, 2010; Sanko, 2017; Singleton, 2020).

to develop affordable, computerized simulators that mimic the body's physiology and react to external interventions (Aebersold, 2018). Several high-fidelity simulators have been developed for medical and nursing education since the middle of the last century, including SimMan, Noelle, and others, making simulated scenarios more realistic (Herrera-Aliaga & Estrada, 2022). With technological advances, SBE has grown to encompass learners from all parts of the globe through online virtual simulation programs and has started to take a step toward virtual reality, allowing the learner to become fully immersed in a scenario.

Despite the widespread use and acceptance in prelicensure nursing education, a gap still exists, proving that SBE positively impacts patient outcomes. Moreover, the effectiveness of SBE in APN programs has a long way to go. However, research is robust, and continued efforts to refine and understand its use can lead to discoveries on how it can impact patient outcomes (Sanko, 2017).

SIMULATION: ENHANCING EDUCATION AND PRACTICE

Nurses are expected to be proficient clinical decision-makers, skilled in holistic health care, and work within interprofessional and multidisciplinary teams to achieve quality and safe patient outcomes (Ayaz & Ismail, 2022; Nickerson & Pollard, 2010). Conducting realistic simulations not only assists with professional skill development and refinement but can also identify gaps in system processes that can lead to harmful patient outcomes (Holtschneider & Park, 2019). Furthermore, concepts, including emotional intelligence, mindfulness of patient care, skilled communication, and effective teamwork have become "buzzwords" in health care settings. These nontechnical skills require learner engagement and reflection that can be fostered by the interactive environment simulation offers (Holtschneider & Park, 2019).

Simulation provides an opportunity to translate knowledge into the practical application of technical and nontechnical skills in a staged learning environment designed to accept and learn from human errors (Campbell et al., 2021; Nye et al., 2019). The uniqueness of simulation in health care is its ability to be adjusted to meet the defined objectives. This can range from simple scenarios for the learner to perform technical skills to complex situations including mass casualty drills for team disaster training (Primeau & Benton, 2021). Educational simulations can be created to expose learners to a multitude of clinical situations in which the experience is controlled, predictable, standardized, and reproducible, which can result in measurable outcomes (Ayaz & Ismail, 2022).

Nursing schools, health care systems, health care credentialing bodies, and professional health care organizations recognize the impact of simulation, making the practice broadly acceptable.

Food for Thought

Does your place of work conduct simulations? What team dynamics or system processes could simulations identify? How can simulation be used to fix those identified issues?

Prelicensure Nursing Programs

Participating in direct patient care during nursing school has been the foundation for prelicensure nurses to acquire the essential concepts of communication, interprofessional collaboration, and critical thinking (AACN, 2021). Undergraduate nursing education has embraced the positive qualities simulation can offer to the learner, patients, and health care systems. Universities offering prelicensure associate degrees in nursing (ADN), bachelors of science in nursing (BSN), and registered-nurse-to-BSN programs have adopted simulation pedagogy. In 2014, the National Council of State Boards of Nursing (NCSBN) released the results of a revolutionary study, *The National Simulation Study*, which supports the substitution of quality simulations for up to 50% of clinical hours for prelicensure nursing students (Alexander et al., 2015). The NCSBN recognized that well-designed simulations can provide learners with quality, consistent, and replicable clinical experiences that can enhance critical thinking within a competency-based curriculum (Anderson et al., 2019; Alexander et al., 2015).

The revised *Essentials: Core Competencies for Professional Nursing Education* by the American Association of Colleges of Nursing (AACN) promotes using simulation experiences in prelicensure programs to augment clinical learning and agrees these experiences are complementary to direct care opportunities (AACN 2021). The majority of the current research on simulation efficacy in nursing has been conducted at the prelicensure level. Positive outcomes identified include student satisfaction, increased self-confidence, improved critical thinking, clinical reasoning, communication, and clinical performance. Furthermore, recent studies have demonstrated similar outcomes for APN students (AACN, 2021; Anderson et al., 2019; Campbell et al., 2021; Nye et al., 2019).

Advanced Practice Nursing Programs

APN programs' simulation adoption has been slower than their prelicensure and medical counterparts yet face similar challenges. The belief the apprenticeship model is the "gold standard" for clinical learning has little empirical data to support its continuation as the only way to acquire clinical hours (Anderson et al., 2019; Campbell et al., 2021). Similar to simulation use in prelicensure nursing programs, the revised AACN *Essentials* endorse clinical learning experiences that can be accomplished through diverse methodologies, including simulation, to assist graduate nurses in becoming proficient in the outlined nursing competencies (AACN, 2021). APN accreditation and certification bodies, the National Organization of Nurse Practitioner Faculties, and the National Task Force for Quality Nurse Practitioner Education endorse simulation as an addition to the minimum direct patient contact hours. Unfortunately, they do not allow direct substitution of clinical hours, believing more rigorous evidence is needed to support the simulation outcomes in the APN population (Lioce et al., 2020; Nye et al., 2019). This recommendation is reasonable; however, the educational climate has changed, due to faculty shortages, inadequate clinical sites, and limited preceptor pools.

Clinical opportunities for APN students have diminished throughout the years, as research has noted the increasing competition for placement spots with medical doctors, physician assistants, and doctors of osteopathy (Anderson et al., 2019; Mason Barber & Schuessler, 2018). Furthermore, current health care reimbursement models, clinical sites, and preceptors facing mounting pressure in maintaining high productivity levels interfere with the time involved in professionally training APN students (Anderson et al., 2019). The strain on preceptors and clinical sites produces inconsistencies in clinical learning experiences and generates newly graduated APNs who are not fully prepared to practice.

SBE can bridge the transition to practice but requires collaboration between educators, students, health care organizations, and credentialing agencies (Anderson et al., 2019; Ayaz & Ismail, 2022). Graham, Knopp, and Schubert (2023) reported on the longitudinal outcomes and qualitative reflections of integrating a scaffolding simulation model into the APN curriculum. Over 1 year, APN students encountered 10 simulation scenarios that paralleled the didactic content. Although the sample size was small ($n = 23$), the pilot study reports that APN students recognized their knowledge gaps, began to create their workflow, acquired elevated confidence, and had an appreciation for a glimpse of what their future work environment might be all before setting foot in a clinical site (Graham et al., 2023). Similar SBE activities in APN education and professional development can guide their transformation into a diagnostic role while building upon their unique perspective of current and past experiences with patient-centered care (Campbell et al., 2021; Graham et al., 2023). As APN students reflect on their current nursing practices in simulation, they begin to recognize where the prior experiences fit into their future professional role; therefore, critical thinking advances and newly gained knowledge is transferred to understanding the complex role of the professional APN in the health care system (Campbell et al., 2021; Graham et al., 2023; Nye et al., 2019). Currently, over 140 APN North American programs have incorporated simulation as a formative evaluation for applying

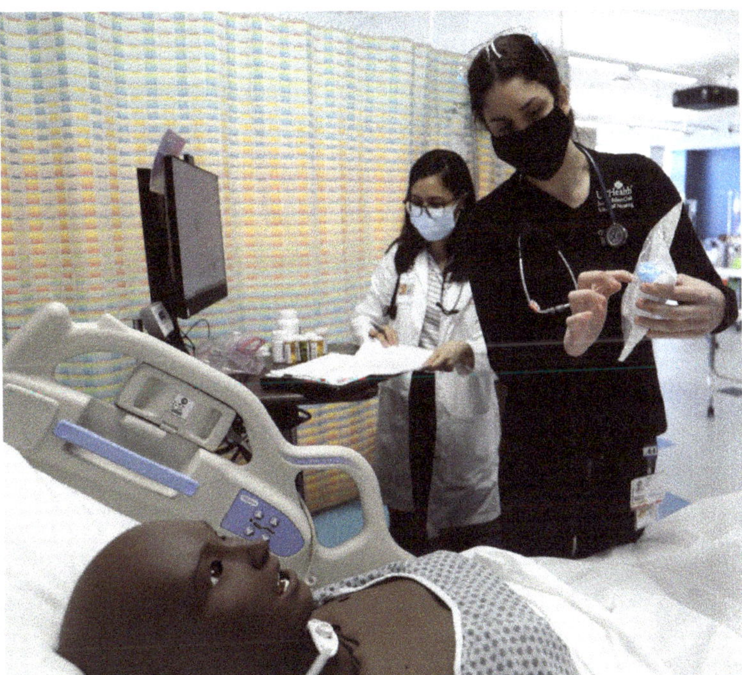

FIGURE 4.4 Advanced practice nursing student (white coat) and prelicensure nursing student (navy blue scrubs) educating a patient (manikin) on a lab collection test.

their skills, a summative evaluation for measuring competencies, and objective structured clinical examinations (OSCEs), not as a teaching pedagogy (Anderson et al., 2019; Nye et al., 2019). Figure 4.4 shows an example of intra-professional simulation where prelicensure students work alongside APN students in a simulated clinical environment.

Food for Thought

As a practicing APN or APN student, what type of simulation scenario or experience would you like to partake in before entering clinical?

Continued Professional Development

Health care professionals must consistently demonstrate professional development by improving their knowledge base, skills, and patient outcomes by remaining relevant to the rapid transformation of health care (Maxworthy et al., 2023). Career-long learning is essential to evolve professional growth and advance the discipline of nursing (AACN, 2021). Moving toward a safer health care system and advancing technology, simulation techniques can be used to refine and introduce skills for advanced learners and create interprofessional team training activities to transform the health care environment (Holtschneider & Park, 2019).

High-quality simulations are ideally suited to provide hands-on, innovative learning and immediate feedback to health care professionals to meet the needs of continuing professional development (CPD) required by their board-certifying bodies (Maxworthy et al., 2023). Simulation-based continuing education offers learners increased levels of interactivity that allow for repeated practice of new skills. Anesthesiologists, obstetricians, and emergency room physicians note the value of simulation and its utility in improved decision-making and testing out new protocols (Forristal et al., 2021). Many hospitals have implemented immersive simulations combined with team strategies and tools to enhance performance and patient safety (Team STEPPS) to focus on leadership and team training to improve patient outcomes (Aebersold, 2016). APNs practicing in ambulatory settings are at a disadvantage, as most of their clinical practice sites are not regulated by hospital systems, so simulation-based continuing education is not readily available and opportunities for interactive continuing education must be sought after.

As future leaders in health care, APNs can prepare themselves to become professional development specialists and become familiar with simulation techniques and how they can be used to achieve educational endeavors. Understanding simulation theory, methodology, and outcomes empowers APNs to advocate for its use in career-long learning and multidisciplinary team training (Holtschneider & Park, 2019). By turning theory into application in a safe environment, practitioners become safe, vigilant, and reflective practitioners, who aim for excellence in quality patient care and proficiency in competencies (Anderson et al., 2019; Nye et al., 2019).

THEORETICAL FRAMEWORKS

Utilizing learning theories to support the objectives and goals of simulation experiences is essential to designing, assessing, and implementing learning experiences. Multiple learning and self-efficacy theories support simulation pedagogy, including Kolb's experiential learning cycle, Knowles's adult learning theory, and Schön's "the reflective practitioner" theory.

Kolb's Experiential Learning Theory

David Allen Kolb's experiential learning cycle is the most prominent theory used as a conceptual framework for simulation programs. Kolb emphasizes that creation of knowledge is a result from experience. Simulation provides immersive environments, allowing multisensory learning that utilizes emotions and effective feedback, which promotes long-term learning (Herrera-Aliaga, 2022; Maxworthy et al., 2023). Kolb's learning cycle consists of four parts (Figure 4.5): concrete experience, reflection, abstract conceptualization, and active experimentation. After participants complete the simulation (concrete experience), debriefing (active reflection) encourages participants to draw generalizations and conclusions based on their observations and performances to form abstract concepts. The concepts should then influence their actions in repeat simulations (active experimentation); however, this step is often omitted, due to time and resources (Ayaz & Ismail, 2022; Maxworthy et al., 2023).

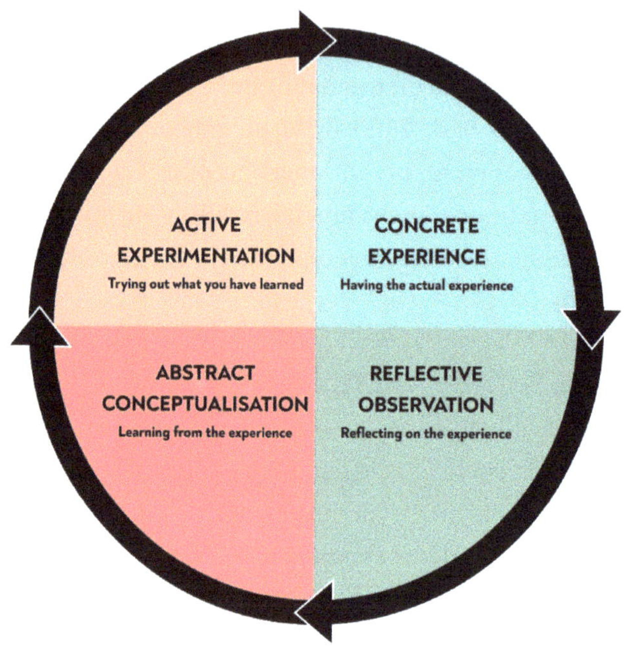

FIGURE 4.5 Kolb's experiential learning cycle.

Knowles' Adult Learning Theory

Malcolm Knowles's adult learning theory (Figure 4.6) states adults are self-directed learners and enter simulations to change their behaviors, skills, and/or knowledge level. Learners must believe there is a benefit to themselves before engaging in educational activities. In addition, Knowles's theory appreciates one's first-hand experiences should be incorporated into the simulation and during debriefing to augment learning (Lioce et al., 2020).

The Reflective Practitioner Theory

Donald A. Schön's "the reflective practitioner" theory supports learning through two types of guided self-reflection: reflection in action (i.e., thinking on your feet) and reflection on action (thinking about previous experiences). Reflection is the critical appraisal of an experience the learner uses to understand their actions,

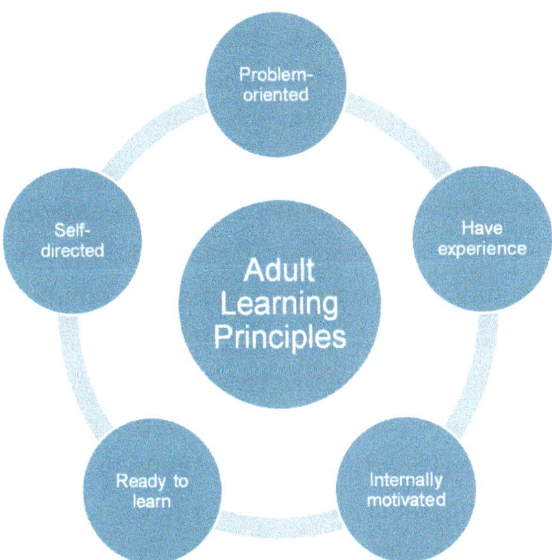

FIGURE 4.6 Knowles's adult learning theory.

meanings, and outcomes, thereby gaining new knowledge that can be applied in future experiences (Cadorette et al., 2023). Learning by doing is essential for developing critical reasoning and clinical judgment skills, whereas reflecting on an experience allows individuals to think about what could have been done differently to achieve similar or better outcomes. This theory complements simulation in nursing education by allowing students to reflect on their practices in a safe, facilitated environment (Cadorette et al., 2023; Lioce et al., 2020). Additional theoretical frameworks used to create simulated-based education include Bandura's social learning theory, deliberate practice theory, Miller's pyramid of professional competence, and Bloom's revised taxonomy (Lioce et al., 2020).

BENEFITS AND LIMITATIONS OF SIMULATION IN NURSING

Nursing schools have been facing a growing shortage of clinical placements for both prelicensure and APN programs, and these shortages have worsened due to the COVID-19 pandemic (Aebersold, 2018; Chan et al., 2021). Given the diminished number of clinical sites for direct patient care and a shortage of nursing faculty, combined with the skills, knowledge, and competencies required to be learned by students, simulation can be a cost-effective approach to student teaching (Bastable, 2021). There are many benefits of simulation in nursing education. Simulation allows students to practice their technical, diagnostic, and nontechnical skills without harming themselves or others. Furthermore, it allows faculty to act as role models, foster peer mentoring, and introduce learners to rare clinical cases to enhance knowledge acquisition (Anderson et al., 2019; Nye et al., 2019). Finally, simulation has become effective in improving team behaviors in interprofessional education (Nye et al., 2019). On the other hand, high-fidelity simulations can be costly and may consume a considerable amount of faculty time and resources in planning and coordination (Campbell et al., 2021; Nye et al., 2019). Table 4.2 summarizes the benefits and limitations of simulation in nursing education (Anderson et al., 2019; Ayaz & Ismail, 2022; Munday, 2022).

Large admission size, lack of financial support, simulation staff, faculty knowledge and training, time commitment, and availability of laboratory space are some of the most significant barriers one might encounter when incorporating simulation into an already-loaded curriculum (Campbell et al., 2021; Nye et al., 2019). There are also no clear guidelines for determining faculty workload for incorporating simulation into an APN program (Nye et al., 2019). Some additional barriers include the lack of standardized definitions, guidelines, and evaluation tools for competency based education using simulation and educator preference for traditional methods of didactic instruction and overactive learning strategies (Lioce et al., 2020).

TABLE 4.2 Major Benefits and Limitations of Simulation

Benefits	Limitations
Improves patient safety	Can be costly (depending on the type of resources utilized)
Improves participant interpersonal communication and empathy	Resource intensive—faculty facilitators, time, planning, and supplies
Improves self-confidence and reduced anxiety among learners	Unable to replicate all the elements of a clinical situation
Offers standardized experiences to all students	Requires nursing faculty trained in simulation
Provides a platform where student competencies can be demonstrated and validated in an efficient manner	Can cause students to learn incorrect information if simulation is of poor quality
Offers avenue for students to actively engage in managing specific patient and family situations	High maintenance—requires dedicated space
Provides opportunities for interprofessional education	Simulation equipment (simulators, monitors, etc.) can be very fragile
Provides a safe environment for integration and application of knowledge	Students may not be fully engaged in the simulation and may not learn from their mistakes
Allows for student reflection on practice choices and translation of knowledge	Dedicated and exclusive faculty may not be available
Provides opportunities to practice critical thinking and enhance skills	Learner-specific individualized teaching not possible
Provides an opportunity to practice nontechnical skills, such as cultural humility, communication, collaboration, and handover	Limited research on clinical skill acquisition and transfer from simulation to clinical environment

NAVIGATING SIMULATION

Classification of Simulation

Classification of simulation in nursing education is based on how interactive the simulator is with the learner and how closely the simulation imitates the real situation for skill performance. "Fidelity," or the realism of the simulations, is described along a continuum from low fidelity to high fidelity, based on the degree to which they approach reality (Jeffries et al., 2016; Sharma et al., 2022). Table 4.3 provides a description, advantages, and disadvantages of each type along with some common examples.

TABLE 4.3 Simulation Classification

Type of Simulation	Description	Advantages	Disadvantages	Examples
Low Fidelity	Involves the practice of one or two basic skills. It is not interactive and has a low level of realism. This simulation type is used to build knowledge.	Easy to construct and less expensive than other simulations	Students can only perform one skill at a time	Wound task trainer for wound management; plastic model arm to learn venipuncture
Medium Fidelity	More technologically sophisticated—more realistic. It is used to build competence.	More realistic and allows more opportunities for learning	Does not impart real practical skills	Full-body manikins that mimic patients with breath sounds, heart sounds, but chest does not rise
High Fidelity	Most realistic with maximum interaction of learners in a realistic environment. This type is used to build performance and action.	Extremely realistic and provides a high level of interactivity and realism	The most expensive and high maintenance	Full-body computerized manikins, standardized patients, virtual reality, and so on

Simulation Modalities

Simulation in health care is considered an activity or event replicating a real clinical situation, utilizing one or a combination of modalities, including role-play, task trainers, simulated manikins, standardized patients, and computer or virtual simulation programs (Ayaz & Ismail, 2022; Herrera-Aliaga & Estrada, 2022; Maxworthy et al., 2023; Nye et al., 2019). Table 4.4 provides a summary of each modality along with the pros and cons of utilizing it in SBE.

TABLE 4.4 Five Dimensions of Simulation Modalities

Type	Definition	Examples	Pros	Cons
Partial-Task Trainers	Representation of portion of human body to develop specific tasks	• CPR dolls • Multivenous IV and injection arms • Pelvic Mentors	• Portable, • static, or wearable • Integration with simulations	• Storage space • Maintenance • Cleaning after use
Role-Playing	Assuming the attitudes and actions of another in a make-believe situation to understand a different point of view	• Student–student interactions • Teacher–student interactions • SP–student interactions	• Cost-effective • Interactive • Can be used with or without equipment • Low stress	• Limited realism is limited • Benefits from trained facilitators • Not seen as "real" or "just a game"
Simulated Manikin	Programmed or operated life-size manikins	• Laerdal SimMan3G • Gaumard • Victoria Birthing Simulator	• Sense of realism • Safe practices • Multifunctional	• Resource intensive • Equipment can malfunction • Expensive • Routine maintenance • Requires programing/ running
Simulated Participant (Standardized Patients)	Volunteers/ actors employed to take the role of the patient	• Scenario-based simulations	• Interactive • Reactive • Heightened Realism • Readily available • Easily implemented	• Costly • Requires training
Electronic/ Virtual Programs	Computer "game" or educational software	• VSim • ShadowHealth • Virtual or augmented reality	• Interactive • Reactive • Mobile • Immersive • Cost-effective • Combined with manikins	• Requires software/ internet • Nontactile learning

In the most basic form of simulation, partial-task trainers are anatomical models used to practice technical skills, including suturing, pelvic exams, blood draw, and injections. These forms of simulation provide opportunities for deliberate practice-repetition of psychomotor or cognitive learners can achieve at their own pace (Ayaz & Ismail, 2022). Task trainers (Figures 4.7 and 4.8) can be integrated into complex simulations to allow students to perform additional skills one could not perform on a simulated participant or manikin (Maxworthy et al., 2023; Nye et al., 2019).

Manikins are designed to replicate the human form and many of its physiological functions. Low-fidelity manikins can help teach specific skills, including two-dimensional displays, static models, and some partial-task trainers (e.g., CPR training dolls) (Maxworthy et al., 2023). High-fidelity manikins are computer-controlled full-body manikins that can closely replicate a patient's physiology, anatomy, and responses, including lung sounds, palpable pulses, and voice response, and can be programmed to respond to appropriate interventions (Maxworthy et al., 2023).

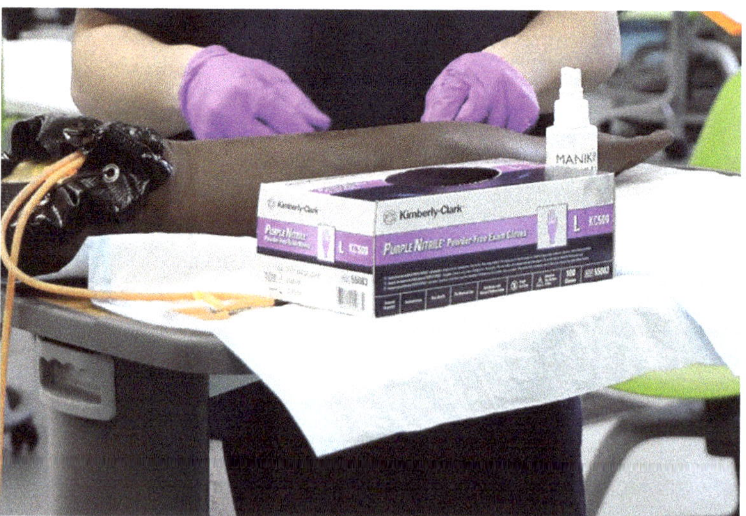

FIGURE 4.7 Task-trainer arm to allow practice of intravenous insertion and blood draws.

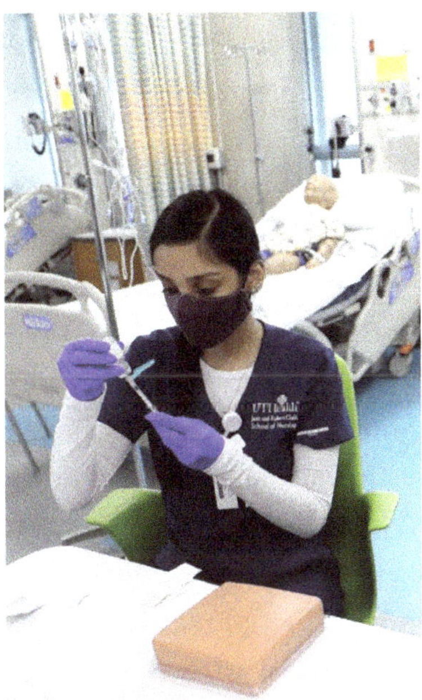

FIGURE 4.8 Injection pad to practice Intramuscular and subcutaneous injections for medication administration.

Virtual technology is utilized where virtual patients are depicted on a computer screen. These dynamic simulations use immersive clinical environments ranging from prehospital environments to community settings. Clinical virtual simulation creates interaction and immediate feedback for the learner. This can result in the learner improving upon several competencies, including clinical skills, critical thinking, and decision-making (Padilha et al., 2019). This form of simulation is gaining popularity in nursing education and has been shown to improve student satisfaction with learning (Padhilha et al., 2019).

UTILIZING SIMULATED PARTICIPANTS

"Simulated participant" (SP) is the universal term for all human role players within SBE who have been properly trained to portray a role consistently. The inclusion of SPs provides significant value in incorporating nontechnical skills, including empathy, patient and family education, communication, and shared decision-making, into an SBE (Cowperthwait, 2020; Maxworthy et al., 2023). In designing simulations for APN training, utilizing simulated participants as patients would be the ideal choice. It can be a cost-effective effort, as it offers the realism of meeting, diagnosing, and treating patients within an outpatient setting.

The best way to replicate a human is with a human (Mason-Barber & Schuessler, 2018). Participants in SBE with SPs value patient-centered feedback, improve their ability to communicate, increase awareness of legal and ethical principles in health care, and gain confidence (Cowperthwait, 2020).

The decision to include SPs within APN simulation is fully supported by the AACN (2021) as a viable adjunct to preceptorship and asserts it would be beneficial to APN education (Figure 4.9). Simulation design that includes the use of SPs should follow established policies and procedures in concordance with the Association of SP Educators Standards of Best Practice and the Healthcare Simulation Standards of Best Practice (HSSOBP) to protect SPs' physical and psychological safety (Cowperthwait, 2020; Maxworthy et al., 2023). Physical safety includes needle safety, air quality, and body mechanics. Psychological safety can be produced by providing the SP with a detailed description of the simulation and their role to identify potential emotional conflicts

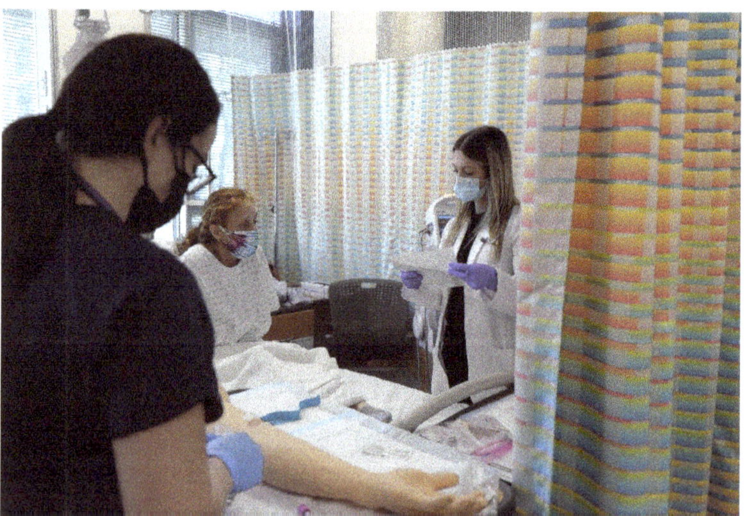

FIGURE 4.9 Advanced practice nursing student (white coat) interviewing a patient (standardized patient) about her symptoms and a prelicensure nursing student (navy blue scrubs) performing a blood draw.

and allow them to opt out if necessary (Cowperthwait, 2020). In addition to role portrayal, SPs can receive training to provide feedback to students regarding their perception of care as the "patient," missed opportunities for communication, or evaluation by student (Mason-Barder, 2017).

METHODS

There are several types of simulation delivery methods. Table 4.5 details some notable methods for conducting simulation and a brief description of each. Many of these methods are used in APN education today.

TABLE 4.5 Methods of Conducting Simulation

In Situ Simulation	Simulation conducted in functional work environment utilizing actual patient or hospital equipment to learn about patient care processes, optimize teamwork and improve patient outcomes
Mobile Simulations	Use of a mobile simulation vehicle or in situ environment to bring medical simulation training to providers to meet the demand of formalized training
Hybrid Simulations	A combination of simulation modalities (e.g., SP for communication and task trainer for skills) to enhance realism and increase the complexity of the scenario
Escape Room Simulations	An immersive learning environment designed in the form of an escape room, where learners encounter a sequence of clues that guide them through a progressive series of assessments and interventions. A completed puzzle helps them "escape." This method promotes learning through teamwork and problem-solving.

(*Continued*)

TABLE 4.5 Methods of Conducting Simulation (*Continued*)

Boot Camps	Intensive courses designed to expose learners to a set of cognitive, technical, and behavioral skills required to lead and manage both common and infrequent issues and crises
Simulation-enhanced Interprofessional Education	Rnables learners from different health care professions to engage in a simulation-based experience to achieve shared objectives and outcomes.
Virtual simulation	An interactive reality technology that creates and mimics real-world patient care encounters. Methods include virtual reality (VR), augmented reality (AR), and virtual standardized patients (VSP).
Unfolding case study	Uses a story format to show how a case evolves and requires learners to apply clinical decision-making that may impact the progression of the case
Distance and Online (Telepresence)	Simulation experiences delivered via an online platform or telepresence such as robotics especially for remotely located learners
Intra-professional simulation	Enables learners from same profession but at different levels (e.g. BSN and APRN students) to engage in a simulation-based experience to achieve shared objectives and outcomes

Note. Adapted from Maxworthy et al., 2023; LaManna et al., 2019; Lioce et al., 2020.

DESIGNING SIMULATION: WHAT TO CONSIDER

Well-designed, structured simulation can offer consistent, measurable educational opportunities and clinical experiences for learners to function as APNs that may not be achievable in clinical settings (Lioce et al., 2020). Consistent outcomes rely on carefully planned and well-orchestrated simulations that can provide a standardized learning experience to all students and present bassline learning opportunities to demonstrate program-level competencies before graduation (Campbell et al., 2021; Nye et al., 2019). Failure to properly execute simulation can lead to unaccomplished or missing objectives, poor to no learning, and disengagement from participants (Ayaz & Ismail, 2022).

Creating a simulation experience requires a stepwise approach. Before designing a simulation, one must assemble a team of simulation enthusiasts and achieve administrative buy-in before starting the project (Maxworthy et al., 2023). Knowing your learners and conducting a needs assessment to take note of the gaps in education will become the basis for the objectives the simulation is supposed to meet. With the measurable outcomes in mind, a mixture of simulation models and modalities can be explored to best suit the chosen content. The National League of Nursing adopted the Jefferies Simulation Model as a guide to the essential practice and foundational principles for SBE (Cowperthwait, 2020). The six core principles of the Jefferies Simulation Model are context, background, design, educational practices, simulation experience, and outcomes.

"Context" is the purpose, physical location, and evaluation criteria of the learning experience, providing the needed framework for developing simulations. Health Care Simulation Standards of Best Practice (HSSOBP) guidelines created by the INACSL are standards that should act as a guide for health care professionals to integrate, use, and advance simulation-based experiences (SBE) within clinical practice, academia, and research (Maxworthy et al., 2023; Watts et al., 2021). "Background" identifies the goals and expectations of the learner, the resources needed, such as time and equipment, and how SBE integrates within the curriculum (Cowperthwait, 2020). Simulation designs should include planned-out phases, including prebriefing, simulation, and debriefing. The HSSOBP and NONPF have guidelines for each phase of simulation, which educators can use to establish policies and procedures within the APN learning environment (Lioce, 2020). Ideally, SBE should be built on measurable objectives and designed alongside content experts and knowledgeable, certified simulation experts to assist with simulation flow, modality, and fidelity choices. Before implementation, conducting a test run is beneficial (Watts et al., 2021).

Food for Thought

If you were to create a low-fidelity simulation for nurses to improve their IV blood-drawing skills, which type of simulation modality and methodology would you choose? What additional objectives could you add to increase fidelity?

SIMULATION PHASES: PREBRIEFING, DESIGN, AND DEBRIEFING

Prebriefing

Prebriefing is a process that involves preparation and briefing. The process of prebriefing ensures that learners participating in the simulation are prepared for the educational content and aware of the ground rules for the simulation-based experience (INASCL Standards Committee, 2021b). Prebriefing is essential in every simulation and should be conducted before the simulation activity. In the prebriefing, facilitators provide learners with information about the goals and objectives of the specific simulation, instructions for the simulation, background information on the patient or scenario, and data about the setting required to complete the simulation (Lioce et al., 2020). The prebriefing steps allow learners to focus on the critical thinking required by the simulation and are vital for learner success and may also enhance debriefing and reflection.

The INASCL Standards Committee (2021b) has divided the prebriefing into two distinct components: preparation and briefing. "Preparation" entails placing the learners into a common mental model and preparing them for the simulation-based experience (SBE) educational content. "Briefing" consists of conveying important ground rules for the simulation-based experience. INASCL standards committee has recommended nine criteria (general, preparation, and briefing) to meet the standard for prebriefing in a simulation-based experience.

General criteria necessary to meet this standard include the following:

- The person leading the simulation should be knowledgeable about the scenario and competent in concepts related to prebriefing per HSSBOP guidelines. This includes maintaining professional development through coursework, formal training, and education.
- Prebriefing should be developed according to the purpose and learning objectives of the SBE. Materials should be developed based on the simulation objectives and information should be provided to the learners in advance of the SBE.
- The experience and knowledge level of the simulation learner should be considered when planning the prebriefing.

Preparation criteria include the following:

- Preparation materials should be developed using adult learning theory principles, and based on needs assessment and purpose of the SBE to ensure that learners are prepared for the experience and meet the scenario objectives.

- Preparation materials should be developed according to the purpose and learning objectives of the SBE. The materials may include assigned readings, audiovisual materials, case studies, completion of a pretest or quiz, review of the electronic health record or patient chart, virtual simulation activities or discussion boards.
- Plan the preparation materials delivery before and on the day of the SBE. The learners should be allowed to complete preparation activities before the SBE to reinforce previous learning. Establishing consequences for learners not completing the preparation requirements will ensure learner readiness for simulation.

Briefing criteria include the following:

- Prior to the SBE, the person planning and leading the simulation should convey valuable information to learners regarding expectations, the agenda, and the logistics for the experience. This includes providing information to the learners regarding their involvement and performance. Detailed logistics such as length of the overall simulation, length of each scenario, location of facilities, and agenda for the day should be provided to the learners. Setting realistic expectations regarding the SBE is important.
- A structured orientation to the simulation-based learning environment should be conducted. Learners and faculty should be oriented to their roles and expectations. Orientation to the equipment and technology used such as manikins, task trainers, virtual learning environments should be provided prior to the SBE.
- Establish a psychologically safe learning environment during the prebriefing. Faculty leading the simulation should establish a safe, trusting environment so learners can express their thoughts without any negative consequences (INASCL Standards Committee, 2021b).

According to the simulation guidelines by NONPF, the six key components of prebriefing are: setting the scene, expectations, debriefing, simulation scenario, simulation room orientation, and preparation time (Lioce et al., 2020). These components are similar to the criteria recommended by the INASCL standards committee for prebriefing.

Simulation Design

The INASCL standards committee has proposed a standard for simulation design and the criteria necessary to meet this standard. Simulation-based experiences designed incorporating best practices from adult learning, instructional design, clinical standards of care, and simulation pedagogy are most effective for learners (INASCL Standards Committee, 2021c). SBEs are purposely designed to meet identified objectives and optimize achievement of expected outcomes. Adapting and using a template that includes goals, objectives, prebriefing case information, scripts, and debriefing points is especially important in simulation design. This will enable the faculty and simulation staff to have information to provide consistent, high-quality, and replicable simulations (Lioce et al., 2020).

Debriefing

Debriefing following health care or simulated events has been argued to be the most critical component for gaining new knowledge that can be applied to future situations (Høegh-Larsen et al., 2023; Maxworthy et al., 2023). Debriefing corresponds with Schon's reflective theory and Kolb's second cycle of reflective practice, wherein individuals must intentionally reflect on their concrete experiences based on the actions performed to form new abstract concepts that can then be applied in new situations (Cadorette et al., 2023; Dreifuerst, 2015; Herrera-Aliaga & Estrada, 2022). Debriefing can be either self-led or conducted within a group setting under the supervision of a trained facilitator. It can easily be adapted to a particular point of care the learner has encountered, making the discussion meaningful, purposeful, and specific (Dreifuerst, 2015). Post-simulation debriefing should create an environment for students to reflect on their own innate beliefs and actions to guide their thinking and future behaviors (Ayaz & Ismail, 2022; Dreifuerst, 2015). During debriefing, learners reflecting on their practice and asked how the simulation fits into their knowledge frame will enable the learner to apply the new knowledge and understanding gained in the simulation and apply it to patient care settings (Nye et al., 2019).

Effective debriefing should occur immediately and be conducted systematically by trained faculty in a ratio of 2–3 dedicated debriefing times to one simulation scenario (e.g., a 15-minute simulation should have 30–45 minutes of debriefing). Audio–visual equipment capable of replaying parts of the individual's scenarios can be helpful but is not required (Herrera-Aliaga & Estrada, 2022; Maxworthy et al., 2023; Watts et al., 2021). Some examples of debriefing methods are described in Table 4.6 and typically follow three phases:

- **reaction:** Learners are invited to express their reactions to the experience. Some example questions include the following:
    - "How did you feel about that simulation?"
    - "How do you feel right now after participating in that simulation?"
- **analysis:** Facilitators create a dialogue of how experiences can be generalized to everyday health care and the implications actions can have on patient care. Some example questions include the following:
    - "What could happen if we continue to miss a step in medication verification in a hospital setting?"
    - "What information would the physician need before we ask for additional orders?"

TABLE 4.6 Types of Debriefing Methods Used in Simulation

Debriefing Model	Summary
Dreifuerst's Debriefing for Meaningful Learning	Nursing-specific debriefing model; cultivates reflective thinking through the Socratic questioning of "who, what, where, when, how, and why?" to help students discover the answers to their own questions
Gather, Analyze, Summarize (GAS) Debriefing	Follows the three phases of debriefing in a highly structured format that promotes self-reflection to improve understanding, practice, and future learning
Debriefing With Good Judgment	Seeks to understand actions of the learners through stating observations of actions and general nonjudgmental inquiry as to why the action was or was not a priority or carried out
Plus-Delta	Straightforward, pointing out the positives (plus) and areas needed for improvement (delta)
Promoting Excellence and Reflective Learning in Simulation (PEARLS) Debriefing	Evidence-based, scripted debriefing model that is learner centered, ia collaborative, and encourages a self-directed approach after clinical and simulation events

Note. Adapted from Dreifuerst, 2015; Høegh-Larsen et al., 2023; Maxworthy et al., 2023.

- **summary:** Learners and facilitators summarize topics discussed and their impact on future practice. Some example questions include the following:
    - "How will this experience change the way you interact with your client in clinical?"
    - "As a recap, we discussed the importance of getting into good habits of washing hands before and after touching a patient."

The chosen method of debriefing must be based on the facilitators' objectives of this program, as each method has its own strengths and weaknesses. Educators can use the Debriefing Assessment for Simulation in Health Care (DASH) tool to measure the effectiveness of debriefing from students and facilitators (Maxworthy et al., 2023). Table 4.6 describes the different types of debriefing methods used in simulation.

EVALUATION IN SIMULATION

There are several purposes of simulation evaluation. It can be used to evaluate the simulation design, debriefing portion, simulation experience itself, student behaviors, student learning, and/or outcomes (Adamson et al., 2013; Maxworthy, et al., 2023). Simulation-based experiences support evaluating the learner's knowledge, technical and clinical skills, communication, decision-making, and competencies, such as patient safety and teamwork skills (Arrogante et al., 2021).

Evaluations can be formative, summative, or high stakes. Formative evaluation is meant to foster development and assist learners in progression toward achieving objectives or outcomes. Summative evaluation focuses on measuring outcomes and the extent to which objectives were met and is usually conducted at the end of the program of study (Billings & Halstead, 2019; INASCL Standards Committee et al., 2021a). High-stakes evaluation (OSCEs) is an assessment that has major implications or consequences based on the outcome. This may include progression or grades for the learners (INASCL Standards Committee et al., 2021a). Table 4.7 provides the criteria for the evaluation of the learners.

Formative Evaluation

Evaluation methods should be chosen based on the objectives, outcomes or level of the learner and guided by the type of evaluation:

TABLE 4.7 The INASCL Standards of Best Practice for Evaluation of Learning and Performance

The INASCL Standards of Best Practice for Evaluation of Learning and Performance State:
"Evaluation of learner(s) using SBEs should include the following elements: A. Determine the type of evaluation for the SBE. B. Design the SBE to include timing of the evaluation. C. Use of a valid and reliable evaluation tool D. Evaluator training E. Completion of the evaluation, interpretation of the results and provision of feedback to the learner(s)"

(INASCL Standards Committee et al., 2021a, p. 54).

formative, summative, or high-stakes evaluation. SBEs may be used for learners' formative assessment to facilitate teaching and learning and to monitor progress toward achieving outcomes (INASCL Standards Committee et al., 2021a). They can also be used to develop learners' clinical competencies and assess readiness to enter practice or clinical setting. Appropriate assessment tools need to be used for formative evaluation (INASCL Standards Committee et al., 2021a).

Summative Evaluation

SBEs may be used for summative evaluation to evaluate learning, skill acquisition, and academic achievement after a defined period. Summative evaluation should be done using a valid instrument, SBE-specific interrater reliability, and a standardized format. Trained facilitators, evaluators or S.P.s should be able to provide feedback to the learners at the conclusion of the evaluation regarding achievement of outcomes (INASCL Standards Committee et al., 2021a).

High-Stakes Evaluation

SBEs may be used for high-stakes evaluation to determine competence, gaps in knowledge, skills, behaviors, and/or to identify safety issues (INASCL Standards Committee et al., 2021a). If using SBEs for high-stakes evaluation, learners must have the opportunity to be exposed to various SBES multiple times, including those with summative evaluations. These should be done by trained evaluators using a standardized evaluation instrument that has been previously tested with similar populations (INASCL standards committee et al., 2021a).

EVALUATION TOOLS

Evaluation tools should be based on precise measurement of attainment of learning objectives. The selected tool should provide an unbiased roadmap for the evaluator (Lioce et al., 2020). The INASCL website has a repository of instruments used in simulation research and is categorized based on multiple domains, such as skill performance, learner satisfaction, knowledge/learning, debriefing, and others. These can be accessed at https://www.inacsl.org/repository-of-instruments; however, there are limited tools for evaluating graduate-level simulations (Nye et al., 2019). The NONPF simulation committee recommends more evidence-based research in advancing the science of APN simulation, including evaluation tools.

MOVING FORWARD WITH SIMULATION IN ADVANCED PRACTICE NURSING EDUCATION

The COVID-19 health care crisis put an additional strain on the nation's frontline health care workers, systems, and communities, disrupting traditional learning experiences (Campbell et al., 2021). Advanced practice programs require students to obtain direct patient clinical care hours to fulfill the clinical education requirements. The COVID 19 pandemic presented unique challenges to these programs because of restrictions in many health care settings, where the students obtained their clinical care hours. (McIltrot et al., 2023).

Use of telehealth has surged since the COVID-19 pandemic. Over 28 million Medicare beneficiaries used telehealth during the first year of the pandemic, a dramatic increase from the prior year (Office of Inspector General [OIG], 2022). Barriers to the use of telehealth, including reimbursement for services, were reduced because of the pandemic. The use of telemedicine and telehealth technology is particularly important in APRN education, due to the increase in chronic diseases requiring disease management. This opens up a new model of health care APNs need to be prepared for and simulation can fill the gap from transition to practice.

In response to the pandemic and the reduced number of clinical sites available to obtain clinical hours, simulation guidelines and best practices for nurse practitioner programs were released by NONPF. This document provides essential guidance for APN faculty seeking to create excellence in SBEs (Lioce et al., 2020). The revised AACN Essentials advocates for simulation as a reliable and valid component of clinical education in advanced-level nursing education (Giddens et al., 2022).

Given the challenges faced by APN education, simulation is a viable option to meet the educational needs of APN students. Educators should adhere to the INASCL's Standards of Best Practice for Simulation and the NONPF guidelines as a framework when designing these SBEs. Evidence of clinical outcomes must be documented during these experiences by evaluating changes in knowledge, skills, and behaviors. AACN's new essentials have emphasized the need for competency-based assessment. Well-planned and executed simulation-based experiences provide an excellent platform for students to demonstrate their knowledge, clinical judgment, and skills to advance (Giddens et al., 2022).

CHAPTER SUMMARY

The link between simulation-based training and an increase in patient safety is becoming apparent, making simulation on the verge of becoming an industry-standard in health care education. Simulation is a fundamental strategy for current and future challenges in nursing education. With the focus on competency-based education, institutions offering APN education should invest in robust simulation activities and infrastructure. Simulation-based experiences that follow the standards of best practice and are well planned can enhance learning outcomes. Training programs for faculty should be conducted to incorporate best practices. More research is needed in evaluation tools for simulation in the APN programs. Technological advances in the simulation arena make the current time the most conducive to embracing simulation in APN education.

Simulation in nursing has evolved over the years and is an integral part of nursing education. Educators use simulations to teach skills, enhance learning outcomes, and promote safe patient care. Simulation in APN education has evolved slower than in prelicensure programs, but the importance of simulation is being recognized. There are various types and modalities of simulation that can be effectively implemented. Simulation is guided by multiple theoretical frameworks, such as Kolb's experiential learning cycle. The INASCL standards committee has published standards of best practice that should be utilized when designing simulations. Simulation phases include prebriefing, simulation design, and debriefing. Simulation can be used for formative, summative, or high-stakes evaluation of learners. Appropriate evaluation tools must be used based on learning objectives. With the focus on competency-based education, institutions offering APN education should invest in robust simulation activities and infrastructure. Simulation-based experiences that follow the standards of best practice and are well planned can enhance learning outcomes.

KEY POINTS

- Evolution of simulation in nursing education—from basic skills to advanced skills

- There are national standards for designing simulation
- There are different methods of evaluation considerations in simulation
- Simulation can significantly benefit APRN education

ACTIVITIES

After reading the chapter on simulation and its use in nursing and future for APNs, consider the following questions or discuss them with a partner or colleague:

1. What is the importance of advocating for simulation in APN programs?
2. What role could simulation play in post-licensure continuing education for APNs?
3. How can simulation be utilized in clinic or community settings to enhance population health?
4. What further research is needed to support the consistent use of simulation in APN education to improve clinical competencies and transition to practice?

REFERENCES

Adamson, K. A., Kardong-Edgren, S., & Willhaus, J. (2013). An updated review of published simulation evaluation instruments. *Clinical Simulation in Nursing*, *9*(9), e393–e405. https://doi.org/10.1016/j.ecns.2012.09.004

Aebersold, M. (2018). Simulation-based learning: No longer a novelty in undergraduate education. *OJIN: Online Journal of Issues in Nursing*, *23*(2), 1–13. https://doi.org/10.3912/OJIN.Vol23No02PPT39

American Association of Colleges of Nursing [AACN]. (2021). *The essentials: Core competencies for professional nursing*. https://www.aacnnursing.org/Portals/42/AcademicNursing/pdf/Essentials-2021.pdf

Alexander, M., Durham, C. F., Hooper, J. I., Jeffries, P. R., Goldman, N., Kardong-Edgren, S. S., ... Tillman, C. (2015). NCSBN simulation guidelines for prelicensure nursing programs. *Journal of Nursing Regulation, 6*(3), 39–42. https://doi.org/10.1016/S2155-8256(15)30783-3

Arrogante, O., González-Romero, G. M., López-Torre, E. M., Carrión-García, L., & Polo, A. (2021). Comparing formative and summative simulation-based assessment in undergraduate nursing students: nursing competency acquisition and clinical simulation satisfaction. *BMC Nursing, 20*(1), 1–92. https://doi.org/10.1186/s12912-021-00614-2

Ayaz, O., & Ismail, F. W. (2022). Health care simulation: a key to the future of medical education - a review. *Advances in Medical Education and Practice, 13*, 301–308. doi:10.2147/AMEP.S353777

Bastable, S. B. (2021). *Nurse as educator: Principles of teaching and learning for nursing practice* (6th ed.). Jones & Bartlett Learning, LLC.

Billings, D., & Halstead, J. (2019). *Teaching in nursing: A guide for faculty* (6th ed.). Elsevier.

Cadorette, J., McCurry, M., & Danells Chin, E. (2023). Reflective transition practice model: The new graduate registered nurse. *Nursing Science Quarterly, 36*(3), 282–291. https://doi.org/10.1177/08943184231169763

Campbell, S. H., Nye, C., Hébert, S. H., Short, C., & Thomas, M. H. (2021). Simulation as a disruptive innovation in advanced practice nursing programs: A report from a qualitative examination. *Clinical Simulation in Nursing, 61*, 79–85. https://doi.org/10.1016/j.ecns.2021.08.001

Chan, G., Bitton, J., Allgeyer, R., Elliott, D., Hudson, L., & Moulton Burwell, P. (2021). The impact of COVID-19 on the nursing workforce: A national overview. *Online Journal of Issues in Nursing, 26*(2), 1–17. https://doi.org/10.3912/OJIN.Vol26No02Man02

Cowperthwait, A. (2020). NLN/Jeffries simulation framework for simulated participant methodology. *Clinical Simulation in Nursing, 42*, 12–21. https://doi.org/10.1016/j.ecns.2019.12.009

Dreifuerst, K. T. (2015). Getting started with debriefing for meaningful learning. *Clinical Simulation in Nursing, 11*(5), 268–275. https://doi.org/10.1016/j.ecns.2015.01.005

Forristal, C., Russell, E., McColl, T., Petrosoniak, A., Thoma, B., Caners, K., ... Hall, A. K. (2021). Simulation in the continuing professional development of academic emergency physicians: A Canadian national survey. *Simulation in Health Care: Journal of the Society for Medical Simulation, 16*(4), 246–253. https://doi.org/10.1097/SIH.0000000000000482

Gaba, D. M. (2007). The future vision of simulation in health care. *Simulation in Health Care: Journal of the Society for Medical Simulation, 2*(2), 126–135. https://doi.org/10.1097/01.SIH.0000258411.38212.32

Giddens, J., Douglas, J. P., & Conroy, S. (2022). The revised AACN essentials: Implications for nursing regulation. *Journal of Nursing Regulation, 12*(4), 16–22. https://doi.org/10.1016/S2155-8256(22)00009-6

Graham, A. C., Knopp, A., & Schubert, C. (2023). A scaffolded simulation curriculum: Translating simulation with standardized patient encounters into clinical practice for nurse practitioner students. *Clinical Simulation in Nursing, 77*, 42–50. https://doi.org/10.1016/j.ecns.2023.02.004

Harris, D. (2018). *Crew resource management for automated teammates (CRM-A).* Springer International Publishing AG.

Health Resources and Services Administration [HRSA]. (2022). Hill-Burton free and reduced-cost health care. https://www.hrsa.gov/get-health-care/affordable/hill-burton

Herrera-Aliaga, E., & Estrada, L. D. (2022). Trends and innovations of simulation for twenty first century medical education. *Frontiers in Public Health, 10*, 619769–619769. https://doi.org/10.3389/fpubh.2022.619769

Høegh-Larsen, A. M., Ravik, M., Reierson, I. Å., Husebø, S. I. E., & Gonzalez, M. T. (2023). PEARLS debriefing compared to standard debriefing effects on nursing students' professional competence and clinical judgment: A quasi-experimental study. *Clinical Simulation in Nursing, 74*, 38–48. https://doi.org/10.1016/j.ecns.2022.09.003

Holtschneider, M. E., & Park, C. W. (2019). Simulation and the nursing professional development practitioner: Learning from the past and looking toward the future. *Journal for Nurses In Professional Development, 35*(2), 110–111. https://doi.org/10.1097/NND.0000000000000531

INACSL Standards of Best Practice. (2016). SimulationSM simulation glossary. *Clinical Simulation in Nursing, 12*, S39–S47. https://doi.org/10.1016/j.ecns.2016.09.012

INACSL Standards Committee, McMahon, E., Jimenez, F. A., Lawrence, K., & Victor, J. (2021a). Health Care Simulation Standards of Best Practice™ Evaluation of

Learning and Performance. *Clinical Simulation in Nursing, 58*, 54–56. https://doi.org/10.1016/j.ecns.2021.08.016

INACSL Standards Committee, McDermott, D. S., Ludlow, J., Horsley, E., & Meakim, C. (2021b). Health care simulation standards of best practice prebriefing: Preparation and briefing. *Clinical Simulation in Nursing, 58*, 9–13. https://doi.org/10.1016/j.ecns.2021.08.008

INACSL Standards Committee, Watts, P. I., McDermott, D. S., Alinier, G., Charnetski, M., & Nawathe, P. A. (2021c). Health care simulation standards of best practice simulation design. *Clinical Simulation in Nursing, 58*, 14–21. https://doi.org/10.1016/j.ecns.2021.08.009

Jeffries, P. R., Swoboda, S.M., & Akintade, B. (2016). Teaching and learning using simulations. In D. M. Billings, & J. A. Halstead (Eds.), *Teaching in nursing: A guide for faculty* (pp. 304–323). Elsevier.

LaManna, J. B., Guido-Sanz, F., Anderson, M., Chase, S. K., Weiss, J. A., & Blackwell, C. W. (2019). Teaching diagnostic reasoning to advanced practice nurses: Positives and negatives. *Clinical Simulation in Nursing, 26*, 24–31. https://doi.org/10.1016/j.ecns.2018.10.006

Lioce, L., Conelius, J., Brown, K., Schneidereith, T., Nye, C., Weston, C., & Bigley, M. (2020). *Simulation guidelines and best practices for nurse practitioner programs.* National Organization of Nurse Practitioner Faculties. https://cdn.ymaws.com/www.nonpf.org/resource/resmgr/docs/simulationnewfolder/20201022_sobp_final.pdf

Mason Barber, L. A., & Schuessler, J. B. (2018). Standardized patient simulation for a graduate nursing program. *Journal for Nurse Practitioners, 14*(1), e5–e11. https://doi.org/10.1016/j.nurpra.2017.09.017

Maxworthy, J. C., Epps, C. A., Okuda, Y., Mancini, M. E., & Palaganas, J. C. (2023). *Defining excellence in simulation programs* (2nd ed.). Wolters Kluwer Health.

Munday, R. (2022). Types of simulation in nursing education. *Nurse Journal.* https://nursejournal.org/resources/types-of-simulation-in-nursing-education/

National Task Force on Quality Nurse Practitioner Education. (2016). Criteria for evaluation of nurse practitioner programs. http://www.acenursing.net/resources/NTF_EvalCriteria2016Final.pdf

Nickerson, M., & Pollard, M. (2010). Mrs. Chase and her descendants: A historical view of simulation. *Creative Nursing, 16*(3), 101–105. https://doi.org/10.1891/1078-4535.16.3.101

Nye, C., Campbell, S. H., Hebert, S. H., Short, C., & Thomas, M. (2019). Simulation in advanced practice nursing programs: A North-American survey. *Clinical Simulation in Nursing, 26*, 3–10. https://doi.org/10.1016/j.ecns.2018.09.005

Office of Inspector General. (2022). *Telehealth was critical for providing services to medicare beneficiaries during the first year of the COVID-19 Pandemic.* https://oig.hhs.gov/oei/reports/OEI-02-20-00520.pdf

Padilha, J. M., Machado, P. P., Ribeiro, A., Ramos, J., & Costa, P. (2019). Clinical virtual simulation in nursing education: Randomized controlled trial. *Journal of Medical Internet Research, 21*(3), e11529. https://doi.org/10.2196/11529

Primeau, M. S., & Benton, A. M. (2021). Multilevel disaster simulation in nursing: Lessons learned in undergraduate and nurse practitioner student collaboration. *Nursing Education Perspectives, 42*(3), 188–189. https://doi.org/10.1097/01.NEP.0000000000000602

Sanko, J. (2017). Simulation as a teaching technology: A brief history of its use in nursing education. *Quarterly Review of Distance Education, 18*(2).

Sharma, R., Jelly, P., Vishwas, A., Chadha, L., & Stephen, S. (2022). Modalities and essentials of simulation facility for facilitation of clinical skills to medical and nursing students: Need for the present era. *Journal of Surgical Specialties and Rural Practice, 3*(1), 1–5. https://doi.org/10.4103/jssrp.jssrp_18_21

Singleton, M. (2020). Flashback Friday—Practice makes perfect: The history of simulation. University of Viginia School of Nursing. https://www.nursing.virginia.edu/news/flashback-history-of-simulation/

Watts, P. I., McDermott, D. S., Alinier, G., Charnetski, M., Ludlow, J., Horsley, E., ... Nawathe, P. A. (2021). Health care simulation standards of best practice simulation design. *Clinical Simulation in Nursing, 58*, 14–21. https://doi.org/10.1016/j.ecns.2021.08.009

Watts, P. I., Rossler, K., Bowler, F., Miller, C., Charnetski, M., Decker, S., ... Hallmark, B. (2021). Onward and upward: Introducing the health care simulation standards of best practice. *Clinical Simulation in Nursing, 58*, 1–4. https://doi.org/10.1016/j.ecns.2021.08.006

Image Credits

Fig. 4.1: Sarah A. Tooley, "A bandaging class with leg models at the London Hospital Nurse Training Program," https://www.nursing.virginia.edu/news/flashback-history-of-simulation/, 1906.

Fig. 4.2: Clovis Didier, "Démonstration du pansement sur manikin," 1916.

Fig. 4.4: Courtesy Cizik School of Nursing at UTHealth Houston.

Fig. 4.5: Saul Mcleod, "Kolb's Experiential Learning Cycle," https://simplypsychology.org/learning-kolb.html. Copyright © 2024 by Simply Psychology.

Fig. 4.6: Teaching and Learning Consulting Network, LLC, "Knowles' Adult Learning Theory," https://www.teachingandlearningnetwork.com/adult-learners.html. Copyright © by Teaching and Learning Consulting Network, LLC.

Fig. 4.7: Courtesy Cizik School of Nursing at UTHealth Houston.

Fig. 4.8: Courtesy Cizik School of Nursing at UTHealth Houston.

Fig. 4.9: Courtesy Cizik School of Nursing at UTHealth Houston.

CHAPTER 5

Advanced Practice Nursing's Role in Social Determinants of Health

Kelly Kearney and Carole Mackavey

OBJECTIVES

Upon completion of the chapter, the student will be able to

1. analyze how social determinants of health impact an individual's health
2. differentiate between and give examples of health, community, and social determinants of health
3. define social determinants of health, social needs, and their impact on individual health

QUESTIONS/CHALLENGES

1. Who are the vulnerable populations in your area?
2. How can you help alleviate a few of the social determinants impacting your area's vulnerable population?

INTRODUCTION: WHAT ARE THE SOCIAL DETERMINANTS OF HEALTH

Despite the United States' significant amount of resources, the income inequality gap, poverty rate, and cost of health care have increased tremendously. While access to affordable health care is essential, other contributors to well-being include where an individual is born, grows, lives, learns, works, eats, and ages (Bowen, 2023). Advanced practice registered nurses (APRNs) must know how health outcomes are affected by characteristics outside of medical management. This chapter examines the social determinants of health (SDOHs), vulnerable populations, health disparities, health inequities, and the impact of SDOHs on mental health.

Health is affected by several nonmedical factors, including income, geographical location, access to health care, and environmental circumstances (Bowen, 2023). SDOHs affect the quality of life, overall functioning, and health outcomes (Wakefield et al., 2021). More than 50% of poor health outcomes are related to SDOH factors, such as structural racism, poor living conditions, unstable housing, and food insecurity (Hacker et al., 2022). Addressing SDOH appropriately is necessary for improving health and dismantling longstanding inequities in health rooted in social and economic disadvantages (Artiga & Hinton, 2019, see Table 5.1).

SDOHs significantly impact well-being and quality of life, even more than medications and other treatments. For example, consider a patient frequently readmitted to the hospital for hypertension. The patient can discuss the importance of exercise, following a diet low in sodium, obtaining a good night's rest, and stress reduction; however, they are frequent flyers in the hospital. Instead of questioning why the patient is not taking proper care of themselves, consider other barriers. Do they have stable housing, access to healthy food, a primary care provider, or transportation to the pharmacy to pick up their medication? It is essential to

TABLE 5.1 Social Determinants of Health

Economic Stability	Neighborhood and Built Environment	Education	Social and Community Context	Health and Health Care
Employment	Quality of housing	Language	Discrimination	Health services accessibility
Housing instability	Environmental conditions	Literacy	Social cohesion	Primary care provider accessibility
Poverty	Access to foods supporting healthy eating	Early childhood education	Civic involvement	Quality of care
Food insecurity	Crime and violence	Vocational training	Community engagement	
		Higher education		

Kelly Kearney and Carole Mackavey, "Advanced Practice Nursing's Role in Social Determinants of Health (SDOH)."

assess these areas when deciding treatment options and feasibility. Our responsibility is to ensure that the necessary resources are available and accessible.

SDOHs generally affect communities and reflect structural policies that serve as barriers to optimal health and well-being. Examples of impacted communities include those without a grocery store, lack of transportation systems, unsafe housing, increased incidence of violence, and limited economic opportunities to promote health (Hacker & Houry, 2022). To combat the determinants, it is essential to form multiple partnerships with health organizations, foster a sense of community trust, and advocate for change to advance health promotion. The most critical component is the engagement of the community members impacted by these factors.

Screening for social needs is essential in determining the overall needs of those impacted by SDOHs. These needs are factors that may affect an individual's health. A health care provider can screen for social factors such as housing and food access. The data will then be used to direct care and provide referrals to social workers, community health workers, or community-based organizations providing direct support to meet patients' social needs (Wakefield et al., 2021). Factors impacting SDOHs should be reviewed alongside the treatment plan routinely.

Policy changes are needed to improve critical areas such as food security, stable housing, and reliable transportation. APRNs must work closely with social workers, case managers, and community organizations to address patients with complex social needs (Wakefield et al., 2021). Partnering with public health organizations is crucial for improving socioeconomic and environmental conditions. Nurses are positioned to promote efforts to integrate SDOH data in clinical decision-making to meet patient needs (Tiase et al., 2022).

Food for Thought

APRNs should understand how SDOH data can be helpful within their health care organization. Learning about the policies and procedures related to SDOHs will aid in the understanding of concepts related to population health. Consider the following in your current organization:

1. Identify common social factors impacting health within your patient population.
2. How can you integrate SDOH data into your nursing workflow to improve patient care?
3. What kind of community-based and other social service programs will you implement to assist in caring for these patients?

VULNERABLE POPULATIONS: WHO ARE THE VULNERABLE POPULATIONS?

"Vulnerability" refers to the degree to which an individual or population is unable to anticipate, cope with, resist, and recover from the impacts of negative or traumatic experiences (World Health Organization [WHO], 2017). Health is a shared global responsibility involving equitable access to essential care for all individuals (Soule, 2021). Vulnerable populations are any population whose social factors significantly impact a person's health. Education, employment status, income level, gender and ethnicity, environmental location, age, and sexual orientation create a vulnerability that can result in poor access to health care, poor-quality care, and experiencing poor care outcomes. For example, people with a chronic illness are twice as likely to have poor health outcomes. Many low-income people are members of ethnic minorities and are more likely to have a chronic disease, lack insurance, and have limited access to health care. Fear of discrimination prevents the LGTBQ population from seeking health care (Joszt, 2018). Children and older adults are more susceptible to illness. The growing number of homeless persons and those with mental health problems are also members of vulnerable populations. The deadly triad of war, famine, and disease contributes to the rapidly growing number of people experiencing health inequity. Refugees and migration are adding to the vulnerable population. Vulnerable populations vary between countries and even between regions in the same country. The American Indians on the reservation in the west and migrant workers and immigrants on Texas's southern border are part of the growing population. Refugees from Afghanistan and Ukraine must also be included.

TABLE 5.2 Some of the Vulnerable Populations

Racial and ethnic minorities	Rural residents with poor access
Economically disadvantaged	LGBTQ+ community
Uninsured or underinsured	Certain genders and gender-nonconforming
Those with chronic health conditions, including HIV, mental health conditions, and obesity	Immigrants
Children and youth	Prisoners
Elderly	Sex-trafficked men and women
Homeless	Human-trafficked men and women
Disabled	Certain religious or cultural groups

Note. Adapted from Morris, 2022.

HEALTH DISPARITY VS. HEALTH EQUITY

What Is Health Disparity?

Healthy People 2030 defines a health disparity as

> a particular type of health difference that is closely linked with economic, social, or environmental disadvantage. Health disparities adversely affect groups of people who have systematically experienced greater social or economic obstacles to health based on their racial or ethnic group, religion, socioeconomic -status, gender, age, or mental health; cognitive, sensory, or physical disability; sexual orientation or gender identity; geographic location; or other characteristics historically linked to discrimination or exclusion. (HealthyPeople.gov, 2014)

"Health disparities" are preventable differences in the burden of disease, injury, violence, or opportunities to achieve optimal health experienced by marginalized and socioeconomically disadvantaged populations (Moreno & Chhatwal, 2020). Health disparities often lead to health inequities caused by gaps that are unjust, unnecessary, unfair, and avoidable (Nash, 2022). These inequities are typically based on deep, historical roots produced and sustained by systems that intentionally and unintentionally prevent people from living their healthiest lives. Historically, marginalized groups suffer from discrimination and have social and economic disadvantages (Moreno & Chhatwal, 2020).

Health care disparities result in patients receiving a lower quality of care and poorer health outcomes (Gergely, 2018). Increasing culturally competent care delivered by APRNs can help to address disparities such as structural racism. Structural racism is a system in which institutional practices, cultural representation, and other norms work to reinforce ways to perpetuate racial group inequity (Mensah et al., 2021). It drives the unequal distribution of opportunities and advantages distributed power according to wealth, rights, and education. Nurses can influence health care organizations and policies to close the gap in health disparities by addressing social needs and SDOHs.

"Social disadvantage" is a broad concept encompassing many topics, but it can be summarized as a person or group's societal position (Braverman, 2014). Many barriers exist; social, geographic, political, economic, and environmental factors all create barriers to vaccination; factors such as education, income, institutional racism, gaps in health care access, transportation, and lack of trust were among a few. As a result, Black or African American, Hispanic, Latino, American Indian, and Alaska Native people are less likely to be vaccinated against COVID-19.

So What Is Health Equity?

"Health equity" is when everyone has a fair and just opportunity to be as healthy as possible, and no one is disadvantaged because of long-standing inequities (CDC, 2022). To achieve health equity, obstacles should be removed, disparities eliminated, and determinants of health that adversely affect excluded or marginalized groups should be identified (Braveman et al., 2018). Attaining health equity goes beyond equitable access to quality care. Health is affected by other factors, such as discrimination and income. Decades of literature indicate the impact of social determinants on health outcomes as we still struggle to achieve health equity for all. One of the overarching goals of Healthy People 2030 is the elimination of health disparities linking health equity to health literacy (U.S. Department of Health and Human Services, 2021).

Addressing social needs can improve health equity in health care. The following five areas facilitate the integration of social care into health care: adjustment, assistance, alignment, advocacy, and awareness (NASEM, 2019).

TABLE 5.3 Definitions of Areas of Activities That Strengthen Integration of Social Care into Health Care

Activity	Definition	Transportation-Related Example
Awareness	Activities that identify the social risks and assets of defined patients and populations	Ask people about their access to transportation.
Adjustment	Activities that focus on altering clinical care to accommodate identified social barriers	Reduce the need for in-person health care appointments using other options, such as telehealth appointments.

(Continued)

TABLE 5.3 Definitions of Areas of Activities That Strengthen Integration of Social Care into Health Care (*Continued*)

Activity	Definition	Transportation-Related Example
Assistance	Activities that reduce social risk by assisting in connecting patients with relevant social care resources	Provide transportation vouchers so that patients can travel to health care appointments. Vouchers can be used for ride-sharing services or public transit.
Alignment	Activities undertaken by health care systems to understand existing social care assets in the community, organize them to facilitate synergies, and invest in and deploy them to positively affect health outcomes	Invest in community ridesharing or time-bank programs.
Advocacy	Activities in which health care organizations work with partner social care organizations to promote policies that facilitate the creation and redeployment of assets or resources to address health and social needs	Work to promote policies that fundamentally change the transportation infrastructure within the community.

Note. From NASEM, 2019.

APRNs are in a critical role in assisting in obtaining the goal of health equity; however, proper education, autonomy, and supportive work environments must be provided (Wakefield et al., 2021). There must be a general understanding of the factors that influence overall health. Interventions should address and consider existing structural barriers that may impede health equity work. The population of focus should be historically marginalized groups and those with significant gaps in health outcomes (Wakefield et al., 2021). The nursing profession can assist in building comprehensive programs designed to benefit everyone.

Leveraging Healthy People to Advance Health Equity
Health Equity is the attainment of the highest level of health for all people.
Achieving health equity requires valuing everyone equally with focused and ongoing societal efforts to address avoidable inequalities, historical and contemporary injustices, and social determinants of health — and to eliminate disparities in health and health care.
Objectives
Identify priorities by browsing Leading Health Indicators and other objectives
Compare population-level progress to national targets
Data
Use Healthy People data to track health disparities and inform program and policy development
Resources
Find inspiration by consulting evidence-based resources to use in your community
Review Healthy People in Action stories to learn how others are addressing health equity
Frameworks
Use the Healthy People 2030 framework as a model for program planning
Use the social determinants of health framework to build partnerships across sectors and communicate root causes of health disparities
Definitions
Use the definitions of health equity and health disparities to promote a shared understanding and identify areas for collaborative action to improve health for all
Leveraging Healthy People to Advance Health Equity
Copyright-free
Healthy People 2030

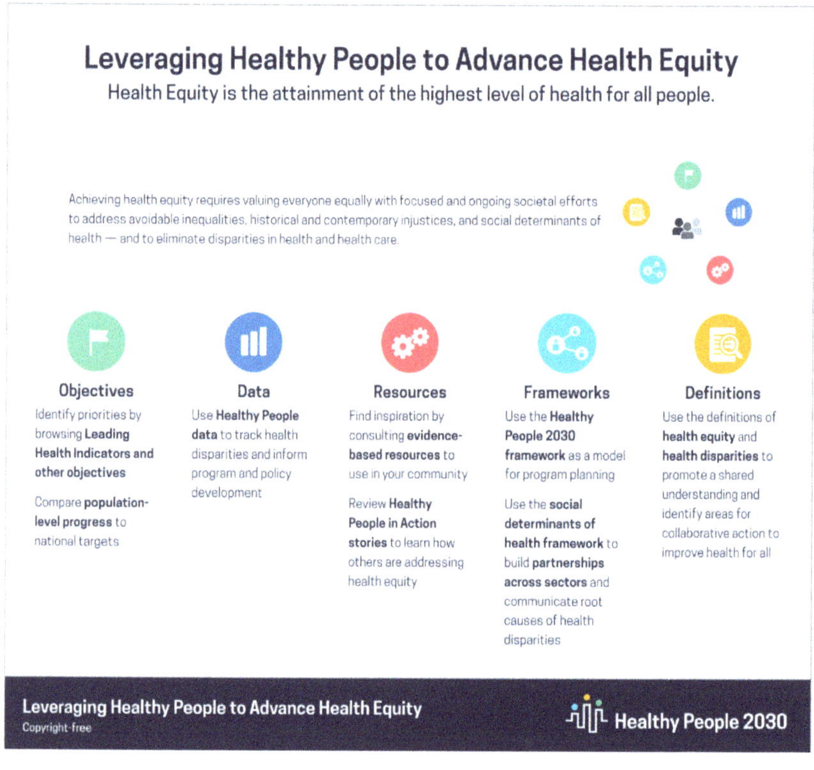

FIGURE 5.1 Achieving Health Equity.

Health equity is an ongoing issue for so many. It is not just about COVID-19; SDOHs impact health care and chronic disease management. Conditions such as heart disease, hypertension, diabetes, cancer screening preventative care, HIV, and hepatitis are all greater risks for people of disadvantaged populations. Only 8% of people in the United States aged 35 and above receive the recommended screenings (Sukhanova et al., 2020). The population is aging, and people are living with multiple chronic diseases.

Food for Thought

How would you address the issue of health disparity to achieve health equity?

ADVANCED PRACTICE ROLE IN CARING FOR VULNERABLE POPULATIONS

Understanding what makes an individual, a group, a community, or a population of vulnerable people is critical when providing care. APNs must consider their biases, prejudices, and stereotypes while working with vulnerable populations. To improve care, APNs can offer their experiences and knowledge in patient care, quality, safety, cost containment, and wellness. Advocating for the vulnerable population, being organizational leaders, and working toward a resolution are all in the role of the APN. Cultural sensitivity and understanding are essential. Partnering with your patient will have a significant impact on the outcome.

The American Academy of Nursing's Edge Runners initiative focuses on nurse-designed models of care and interventions that impact cost and improve health care quality. Programs such as Nurses Improve Care for Health Systems Elders (NICHE) developed geriatric protocols that impacted staffing patterns and reduced preventable complications in the aging population, while other programs addressed the increased rate of homelessness. APNs and nurses contribute to the health care of vulnerable populations in community clinics and nursing homes through innovative, evidence-based, nurse-led clinical models of care (Xue & Intrator, 2016).

Unfortunately, SDOHs are unequal across gender, class, race, sexual orientation, and socioeconomic and minority groups. APNs are uniquely positioned to provide advocacy and education, increase awareness, and improve health care access.

IMPACTS OF SDOHs ON MENTAL HEALTH

Social determinants of mental health are societal problems that inhibit one from experiencing optimal mental health, increasing the risk for poor outcomes among individuals with mental illnesses (Shim & Compton, 2020). Individuals with lower socioeconomic status may report adverse mental health events, including daily stress, perceived loss of control, and anxiety about living situations. Unstable employment and financial strain are linked to increased psychological distress. Lower-income individuals are more likely to experience poor housing conditions, food insecurity, and poorer nutrition related to poor mental health.

Neighborhood characteristics and the perception of safety can also impact mental health. Experiencing or witnessing community violence can increase the risk of depression, anxiety, and post-traumatic stress disorder (PTSD). For example, police killings of unarmed African American males can contribute to an undue amount of anxiety, depression, and paranoia within communities.

The utilization of support programs can increase employment rates and will have a positive impact on overall well-being. Housing programs can increase stable housing, decrease the revolving door of inpatient psychiatric hospitalizations, and stabilize the health services of those experiencing homelessness (Alegría et al., 2018). Incorporating community-based interventions to institute neighborhood trust, increase safety, and diminish violence and crime may lessen mental health inequalities.

Improving social connectedness and inclusion can have a positive impact on mental health. Peer support and partnership with faith-based communities are additional components to improve mental health outcomes (Jeste & Pender, 2022). Perceived emotional support, community belonging, and trust are related to positive mental health outcomes and can be protective against the more common mental health disorders (Alegría et al., 2018). Integrating behavioral health services into primary care can encourage systems to better respond to SDOH of mental health (Jeste & Pender, 2022). A well-planned, comprehensive approach is vital to address the long-term impacts on mental health.

IMPACTS OF SDOHs ON RURAL HEALTH CARE

Rural America is home to roughly 46 million Americans, approximately 72% of the United States (NCSL, 2023), yet those living in rural areas are more likely to experience barriers and challenges to health care access. Low income, poor health literacy, race/ethnicity, sexual orientation/gender identity, environmental issues, and limited transportation are all contributing factors. Modern health challenges, including chronic disease, an aging population, considerable diversity, and existing health disparities, will only contribute to the problem.

The lack of primary care providers in rural and medically underserved areas is not in dispute; however, the solution is. APNs are uniquely qualified to fill the gap in primary care. Many reports show that NPs are significantly more likely than primary care physicians to care for vulnerable populations (Buerhaus, 2018).

COVID-19 created a need for a new definition of APN professional roles. The evidence supporting APNs working areas of care often maintains or improves the quality of care and outcomes for patients. Ortiz et al. (2018) studied the impact of APN-restricted practice versus independent practice in rural health by examining five chronic disease outcomes. Their study found no significant difference between the diseases as well as that the quality of patient outcomes was not significantly impacted by an APN-independent approach. The authors of the study also state that APNs may be the answer to reducing the primary care shortage in rural areas (Ortiz et al., 2018).

CHAPTER SUMMARY

The needs of vulnerable populations must be addressed and valued to foster an inclusive and equitable population. Empowering communities through education, access to resources, and community engagement can significantly reduce health disparities. Focusing on prevention, early intervention, and culturally competent interventions can target the root cause of health disparities. Culturally competent interventions should be developed with consideration of marginalized groups and their specific challenges.

Understanding the unique social determinants that impact vulnerable populations and tailoring health care services to meet their specific needs is pivotal in advancing health equity. Committing to social justice and standing up for human rights can assist in dismantling systemic barriers and minimizing vulnerabilities. Reducing disparities requires a collaborative effort from all to implement strategies.

Social determinants have a profound and lasting impact on health outcomes in various populations. A collaborative and comprehensive approach is required from APRNs, other health care providers, policymakers, and the community to address systemic barriers and health disparities. Each community should consider its unique makeup to determine the most appropriate interventions to improve population health. Recognizing and moving forth initiatives involving SDOHs can assist individuals in attaining their optimal level of health while creating an equitable society.

APRNs are instrumental in championing health equity and combating health disparities. Regardless of their background, all people should have the opportunity to achieve optimal health and well-being. APRNs can build trust within the communities by displaying compassion and using patient-centered approaches that make meaningful contributions to the creation of a health care system that is fair, just, and inclusive for all.

KEY POINTS

- Advanced practice nurses are uniquely positioned to address the SDOHs in their care.
- Culturally competent care is critical to addressing SDOHs and providing effective health care.
- Understanding patients' cultural context allows the practitioner to develop a plan that will better meet the patient's needs.

ACTIVITIES

1. How would you address the concerns of a 55-year-old Hispanic mother of six recently diagnosed with type 2 diabetes, who is worried about how she will afford to make the costly health changes, such as purchasing fresh produce, recommended to her?
2. How would you address the concerns of an African American woman with obesity, who asks you about exercising? She states she can only work out after work but feels unsafe walking around her neighborhood at night.
3. Consider the issue of nutrition when there is limited transportation and your patient lives in a food desert.

REFERENCES

Alegría, M., NeMoyer, A., Falgàs Bagué, I., Wang, Y., & Alvarez, K. (2018). Social determinants of mental health: Where we are and where we need to go. *Current Psychiatry Reports*, *20*, 1–13.

American Academy of Nursing [AAN]. (n.d.). *Transforming America's health system through nursing solutions*. https://www.aannet.org/initiatives/edge-runners

Artiga, S., & Hinton, E. (2019). Beyond health care: The role of social determinants in promoting health and health equity. *Health*, *20*(10), 1–13.

Barnes, H., Richards, M. R., McHugh, M. D., & Martsolf, G. (2018). Rural and nonrural primary care physician practices increasingly rely on nurse practitioners. *Health Affairs, 37*(6), 908–914. https://doi.org/10.1377/hlthaff.2017.1158

Bowen, F. (2023). The ABCs of DEI. AJN *The American Journal of Nursing, 123*(1), 19–20.

Braveman P. (2014). *What are health disparities and health equity? We need to be clear* (129 Suppl 2(2), 5–8). Public Health Reports. https://doi.org/10.1177/00333549141291S203

Braveman, P., Arkin, E., Orleans, T., Proctor, D., Acker, J., & Plough, A. (2018). What is health equity? *Behavioral Science & Policy, 4*(1), 1–14. https://doi.org/10.1353/bsp.2018.0000

Buerhaus, P. (2018). *Nurse practitioners: A solution to America's primary care crisis.* American Enterprise Institute. https://www.aei.org/research-products/report/nurse-practitioners-a-solution-to-americas-primary-care-crisis/

Center for Disease Control. (2020). *Health disparities.* https://www.cdc.gov/healthyyouth/disparities/index.htm#print

Center for Disease Control. (2022). *What is health equity?* https://www.cdc.gov/nchhstp/healthequity/index.html

Garrigues, L. J. (2021). Addressing health inequities in vulnerable populations through social justice. In A. Vermeesch (Ed.), *Integrative health nursing interventions for vulnerable populations.* Springer Nature. https://doi.org/10.1007/978-3-030-60043-3

Gergely, S. (2018). Cultural competency matters. *JONA: The Journal of Nursing Administration, 48*(10), 474–477. https://doi.org/10.1097/NNA.0000000000000654

Hacker, K., Auerbach, J., Ikeda, R., Philip, C., & Houry, D. (2022). Social determinants of health—An approach taken at CDC. *Journal of Public Health Management and Practice, 28*(6), 589–594.

Hacker, K., & Houry, D. (2022). Social needs and social determinants: The role of the Centers for Disease Control and Prevention and Public Health. *Public Health Reports, 137*(6), 1049–1052.

Health Resources and Services Administration. (2022). *Defining rural population.* https://www.hrsa.gov/rural-health/about-us/what-is-rural

HealthyPeople.gov. (2014). *Disparities.* http://www.healthypeople.gov/2020/about/disparitiesAbout.aspx

Jeste, D. V., & Pender, V. B. (2022). Social determinants of mental health: Recommendations for research, training, practice, and policy. *JAMA Psychiatry, 79*(4), 283–284.

Joszt, L. (2018). 5 vulnerable populations in health care. *American Journal of Managed Care.* https://www.ajmc.com/view/5-vulnerable-populations-in-health care

Kaplan, L. (2020). The importance of building a strong, rural NP workforce. *The Nurse Practitioner, 45*(9), 8–9. https://doi.org/10.1097/01.NPR.0000694736.51794.1b

Laurant, M., Harmsen, M., Wollersheim, H., Grol, R., Faber, M., & Sibbald, B. (2009). The impact of nonphysician clinicians: Do they improve the quality and cost-effectiveness of health care services? *Medical Care Research and Review, 66*(6 Suppl), 36S–89S. https://doi.org/10.1177/1077558709346277

Mensah, M., Ogbu-Nwobodo, L., & Shim, R. S. (2021). Racism and mental health equity: History repeating itself. *Psychiatric Services, 72*(9), 1091–1094.

Morris, G. (2022). Working with vulnerable populations as a nurse practitioner. *Nurse Journal.* https://nursejournal.org/resources/nps-vulnerable-populations/#:~:text=Nurse%20practitioners%20can%20advocate%20for,%2C%20health care%20institutions%2C%20and%20communities

National Academies of Sciences, Engineering, and Medicine. (2019). *Integrating social care into the delivery of health care: Moving upstream to improve the nation's health.*

National Conference of States Legislatures. (2023). Agriculture and rural development. https://www.ncsl.org/agriculture-and-rural-development#:~:text=Rural%20America%20makes%20up%2072,with%20manufacturing%2C%20services%20and%20trade

Office of Disease Prevention and Health Promotion. (2022). *Health equity and health disparities environmental scan.* https://health.gov/sites/default/files/2022-04/HP2030-HealthEquityEnvironmentalScan.pdf

Ortiz, J., Hofler, R., Bushy, A., Lin, Y. L., Khanijahani, A., & Bitney, A. (2018). Impact of nurse practitioner practice regulations on rural population health outcomes. *Health Care (Basel, Switzerland), 6*(2), 65. https://doi.org/10.3390/healthcare6020065

Shim, R. S., & Compton, M. T. (2020). The social determinants of mental health: Psychiatrists' roles in addressing discrimination and food insecurity. *Focus, 18*(1), 25–30.

Soulé, I. (2021). Cultural humility. In A. Vermeesch (Ed.), *Integrative health nursing interventions for vulnerable populations.* Springer Nature Switzerland AG. https://doi.org/10.1007/978-3-030-60043-3

Tiase, V., Crookston, C. D., Schoenbaum, A., & Valu, M. (2022). Nurses' role in addressing social determinants of health. *Nursing, 52*(4), 32–37.

Ukhanova, M. A., Tillotson, C. J., Marino, M., Huguet, N., Quiñones, A. R., Hatch, B. A., Schmidt, T., & DeVoe, J. E. (2020). Uptake of preventive services among patients with and without multimorbidity. *American Journal of Preventive Medicine, 59*(5), 621–629. https://doi.org/10.1016/j.amepre.2020.04.019

United States Census Bureau. (2022). Nation's urban and rural populations shift following 2020 Census. https://www.census.gov/newsroom/press-releases/2022/urban-rural-populations.html

U.S. Department of Health and Humans Service (2021). Healthy People 2030 accessed https://health.gov/healthypeople/about/healthy-people-2030-framework#:~:text=Healthy%20People%202030's%20overarching%20goals,and%20well%2Dbeing%20of%20all.

Wakefield, M., Williams, D. R., & Le Menestrel, S. (2021). *The future of nursing 2020–2030: Charting a path to achieve health equity.* National Academy of Sciences

Woo, B. F. Y., Lee, J. X. Y., & Tam, W. W. S. (2017). The impact of the advanced practice nursing role on quality of care, clinical outcomes, patient satisfaction, and cost in the emergency and critical care settings: A systematic review. *Human Resources for Health, 15*(1), 63. https://doi.org/10.1186/s12960-017-0237-9

Xue, Y., & Intrator, O. (2016). Cultivating the role of nurse practitioners in providing primary care to vulnerable populations in an era of health-care reform. *Policy, Politics & Nursing Practice, 17*(1), 24–31. https://doi.org/10.1177/1527154416645539

Image Credit

Fig. 5.1: Healthy People 2030, "Leveraging Healthy People to Advance Health Equity," https://health.gov/healthypeople/priority-areas/health-equity-healthy-people-2030.

CHAPTER 6

Advanced Practice Nursing and Telehealth

Carole Mackavey

OBJECTIVES

Upon completion of the chapter, the student will be able to

1. examine the role of telehealth in modern health care
2. explore the opportunities that telehealth will afford all aspects of medicine in the future
3. distinguish between the various types of telehealth
4. discuss the advantages and disadvantages of telehealth

QUESTIONS/CHALLENGES

1. What are your thoughts on telehealth in general?
2. What are your thoughts on the use of telehealth for the administration of mental health services?
3. What areas of health care do you think would benefit from telehealth?

INTRODUCTION

The impact of COVID-19 on health care and the world, affecting over 18.3 million people worldwide and resulting in over 695,000 deaths (Doraiswamy et al., 2020), will long be remembered. At the onset of the pandemic, more than 50 U.S. health systems already had telehealth or telemedicine programs to allow clinicians to see patients at home (Hollander & Carr, 2020). Technology became a vital tool for managing patients, providing education, and limiting exposure during the pandemic.

Individual states and the federal government regulate telehealth. In 1996, the Institute of Medicine (IOM) defined telemedicine as "the use of electronic information and communications technologies to provide and support health care when distance separates participants" (IOM, 1996, p. 1). Telehealth is simply a tool that allows providers to manage patients without their physical presence in the office. It enables patient data to be transmitted across a long distance, with the original intent of providing care for rural and underserved patients (Balestra, 2018). While telehealth does increase access to health care, for several reasons, some populations may not be able to participate to the same extent as others. For example, for those with limited internet access, one alternative is audio-only telehealth, which does not require broadband access.

DEFINING TELEHEALTH AND TELEMEDICINE

Telehealth uses electronic information and telecommunication technologies to support long-distance clinical health care, patient and professional health-related education, public health, and health administration. Technologies include video conferencing, the internet, store-and-forward imaging, streaming media, and terrestrial and wireless communications (Wijesooriya et al., 2020). Telemedicine uses electronic technology or media, including interactive video conferencing technologies, to diagnose or treat patients, provide remote patient monitoring services, or consult with other health care providers regarding a patient's diagnosis or treatment (Wijesooriya et al., 2020).

This chapter focuses on the pandemic's role in telehealth's growth and the use of telehealth in managing the general population. Nesbit (2012) cited the 2001 IOM report that stated, "Information technology must play a central role in the redesign of the health care system if a substantial improvement in quality is to be achieved" (IOM, 2001, p. 16). There will always be someone who does not have access to new and innovative technology, so disparities will grow. Telehealth can help overcome some presenting disparities (Nesbit, 2012).

In March 2020, the delivery of health care was redesigned. Telehealth is expanding at an alarming rate in hospitals, urgent care, primary care, mental health, and emergency rooms. The U.S. government declared a state of emergency, and many previously enforced barriers to using telehealth were lifted (Kobeissi & Hickey, 2023). The number of telehealth visits increased by 154% during the early period of the outbreak in March 2020 (Koonin et al., 2020).

Telehealth became an invaluable tool for safely and effectively reaching patients during the COVID-19 pandemic. Telehealth decreases the risk of exposure for patients and providers (Wijesooriya et al., 2020). Telehealth was used extensively during the pandemic for diagnosis, treatment, "e-prescribing" medications, and follow-up care (Doraiswamy et al., 2020), mental health services, chronic disease management, and many other specialties. Telehealth bridged the gap, allowing providers to reach rural communities where limited access to health care creates a void in services.

APN education should include technology like telehealth in providing care and the federal rules and regulations governing telehealth practice. The APN role is expanding, and in many places, the traditional face-to-face visit has been replaced by telehealth technologies. The evolution of telehealth and artificial intelligence (AI) in health care has been remarkable, transforming how medical services are delivered and improving patient outcomes. Health care technologies and telepresence are crucial in enhancing patient care, improving medical processes, and enabling remote interactions between health care providers and patients.

Video conferencing allows health care providers to conduct virtual consultations with patients, offer medical advice, and discuss treatment plans. Remote patient monitoring devices collect and transmit health data, enabling continuous monitoring. Additionally, wearable health devices, such as smartwatches and fitness trackers, can monitor various health metrics (Lee & Kim, 2020).

Technologies such as virtual reality (VR) and augmented reality (AR) are being explored in health care for medical training, surgical planning, pain management, and patient education. Telepresence robots designed to replicate a human's presence in a remote location are also in use. These robots are often used to facilitate remote consultations, enabling specialists to meet with patients and collaborate with on-site health care teams. Since about 2010, artificial intelligence (AI) has been used as a support system for health care providers in making more accurate clinical diagnoses and treatment recommendations. AI-powered surgical robots and tools assist surgeons with enhanced precision and minimal invasiveness. They are used in procedures ranging from minimally invasive surgeries to complex interventions and in genomic medicine to analyze individual patient data, genetic information, and environmental factors (ChatGPT, personal communication, August 2023).

Integrating health care technologies and telepresence addresses geographical barriers and enhances health care accessibility, patient engagement, and overall quality of care. The health care industry will likely see even more innovative solutions as technology advances.

TABLE 6.1 The Evolution of Telehealth

Early Beginnings (1960s–1990s)	The concept of telehealth emerged with telephones and early video conferencing to provide medical consultations and advice to patients in remote areas.
Internet Era (2000s–2010s)	With the widespread internet adoption, telehealth expanded to include online platforms, email consultations, and remote monitoring of patient's vital signs. This decade saw the beginnings of electronic health records (EHR) systems.
Mobile Health (mHealth) (2010s)	Smartphones and mobile apps brought about mHealth, enabling patients to access medical information, receive reminders, and interact with health care providers. Wearable health devices also gained popularity for monitoring fitness and health statistics.
Advanced Telehealth (2010s) Present	High-speed internet, improved video conferencing technology, and regulations supporting telehealth reimbursement led to a surge in virtual doctor visits, especially in rural or underserved areas. Remote patient monitoring devices expanded to cover chronic conditions, like diabetes and hypertension.
COVID-19 Impact (2020s)	The COVID-19 pandemic accelerated the adoption of telehealth exponentially. Lockdowns and social distancing measures necessitated remote health care services, prompting patients and health care providers to embrace telehealth solutions.

Note. Adapted from ChatGPT, personal communication, August, 2023.

TYPES OF TELEHEALTH DEFINED

There are four types of telemedicine: real-time (or live video), asynchronous (aka "store-and-forward" or "capture, store, and forward"), remote patient monitoring, and mobile health.

- **real-time:** Videoconferencing technology is used in telehealth to connect two or more people in a live conversation for purposes related to health care delivery or education using cameras, two TVs, a microphone, software, and computer networks, which transmit audio and video data in real time (NONPF, 2018).
- **asynchronous:** This "store-and-forward" technology collects patient data and sends it to the intended destination. Typical store and forward data include radiology and medical imaging, retinal photos, patient physiologic data, electrocardiograms, patient education and symptom survey data, and wound images. Systems collect data at a source and forward it for review, eliminating the need for the provider to meet with the patient to obtain data (NONPF, 2018).
- **mobile health (mHealth):** These systems use live, store, and forward technologies via mobile wireless electronic devices, such as mobile phones or wearable health devices. This format advances health, health care, health information, and education by allowing patients access to health care professionals anytime (NONPF, 2018).
- **remote monitoring:** This form of technology uses sensors and devices that measure physiologic data. Remote monitoring systems collect data at one site and then transfer that data to a device, a centralized monitoring program, or a health care provider for evaluation. Remote monitoring systems use medical equipment (scales, pulse oximetry, stethoscopes, otoscopes,

ophthalmoscopes, etc.) to connect, record, and transmit diagnostic information, such as weight, oxygen saturation, and lung and heart sounds (NONPF, 2018).

TELEHEALTH COMPETENCIES

The Association of American Medical Colleges (AAMC, 2021) developed a set of telehealth competencies designed to add depth to the existing competencies.

The competencies are organized across six domains:

- **patient safety and appropriate use of telehealth:** Clinicians will understand when and why to use telehealth and how to assess patient readiness, patient safety, practice readiness, and end-user readiness.
- **access and equity in telehealth:** To promote equitable access to care, clinicians will understand telehealth delivery that addresses and mitigates cultural biases and physician bias for or against telehealth and that accounts for physical and mental disabilities and non-health-related individual and community needs and limitations.
- **communication via telehealth:** Using telehealth modalities, clinicians will effectively communicate with patients, families, caregivers, and health care team members. They will also integrate the transmission and receipt of information to promote effective knowledge transfer, professionalism, and understanding within a therapeutic relationship.
- **data collection and assessment via telehealth:** Clinicians will obtain and manage clinical information via telehealth to ensure appropriate, high-quality care.
- **technology for telehealth:** Clinicians will have basic knowledge of the technology needed to deliver high-quality telehealth services.

- **ethical practices and legal requirements for telehealth:** Clinicians will understand the federal, state, and local facility practice requirements to meet the minimal standards to deliver health care via telehealth. Clinicians will maintain patient privacy while minimizing risk to the clinician and patient during telehealth encounters, putting the patient's interest first, and preserving or enhancing the doctor-patient relationship.

ADVANTAGES AND DISADVANTAGES OF TELEHEALTH

Historically, barriers to care included the time and distance required to travel to the provider, unreliable transportation, or a complete lack of transportation. Before the pandemic, telehealth services were limited but proved effective in reducing readmission in heart failure patients through early identification of symptoms. Remote monitoring also allowed the providers to adjust treatment regimens (Flodgren et al., 2015; Mahtta et al., 2021).

The COVID-19 pandemic triggered the rapid expansion of telehealth. Patients and providers could interact via telecommunication systems to share information and review current issues. Telehealth improved patient access and extended the geographic reach of the providers (ATA, 2023). Telehealth has been shown to improve cost savings by eliminating patients' travel time, accurate triages, reducing emergency room visits, limiting time away from work, and improving patient outcomes (ATA, 2023; Balestra, 2018; Mahtta et al., 2021). There is a provider shortage in many rural and underserved areas; telehealth is an option that will increase access and improve the timeliness of care (ATA, 2023).

King Dailey et al. (2022) identify telehealth as a cost-effective and efficient way to review symptoms and weight monitoring. A more in-depth assessment was possible with remote cardiac monitoring (implantable and wearable devices; King-Dailey et al., 2022). DeNicola et al. (2020) reviewed 47 articles with 31,967 participants and examined the existing evidence on the effects of remote monitoring and virtual visits on women's health care delivery. They noted improvements in obstetric outcomes, early access to medical abortion services, and schedule optimization for high-risk obstetrics (DeNicola et al., 2020).

In a qualitative study, Nicosia et al. (2021) used telehealth to improve access to care in a Veterans Administration TeleSleep program. The positive airway pressure (PAP) device was remotely monitored. Ninety percent of the participants in the study lived in rural areas. Participants reported that the local clinic was at least 45 minutes away; some were on oxygen, so they could not take public transportation or drive due to Obstructive Sleep Apnea (OSA). Many rural participants in the study opted for video visits. One was quoted as saying it is a "wonderful innovation." The patients' experiences were positive, reducing travel burden and improving quality of life outcomes (Nicosia et al., 2021). Telehealth is also being used in dermatology and mental health.

Medical education has also been enhanced through video conferencing. Project Extension for Community Healthcare Outcomes (ECHO) from the University of New Mexico trains and supports primary care providers in managing various conditions. ECHO offers educational classes and consults worldwide, bringing scarce clinical expertise to rural or remote locations (AHRQ, 2023).

With the onset of COVID-19, telehealth visits increased by 154% (Koonin et al., 2020). By April 2020, nearly all primary care physicians (97%) used telemedicine to treat patients (ATA, 2021). Initially, telehealth was used for remote screening and management of COVID-19. As the pandemic progressed, social distancing became the new normal, and many people stopped going to their primary care providers for follow-up visits for chronic conditions. Telehealth was highly regulated before the pandemic (Kobiessi & Hickey, 2023). The U.S. government's declaration of a national state of emergency resulted in waivers being issued to remove barriers to the use of telehealth. The administration initially planned to end the public health emergency on May 11, 2023. The Consolidated Appropriations Act of 2023 has extended the telehealth flexibilities initiated during COVID-19 through December 31, 2024.

Food for Thought

1. Does the use of telehealth contribute to dehumanization by virtualizing patients and care and focusing on measurement?
2. Will the disadvantages of telehealth foster health disparity, and if so, why?

Disadvantages

There is concern among some that telehealth minimizes the patient–provider relationship, the problem of patient digital literacy, and some individuals' lack of access to computers, tablets, smartphones, and other devices. Many underserved communities do not have the means to participate in telehealth. Some of the issues reported by patients included the lack of stable internet access and a suitable smart device for accessing the charts. Lack of insurance coverage for telehealth may also be an issue. Other issues include a lack of housing or private space to participate in virtual visits; a limited number of local providers who offer telehealth practices; language barriers, including oral, written, and signed language; and a lack of adaptive equipment for people with disabilities. COVID-19 highlighted vast racial, social, and economic inequities. These inequities will continue to exist in telehealth and must be addressed.

APN PRACTICE

Before beginning a telehealth service, ensure the technology is in place and works. Explain to the patient how to use the technology. Provide all components of patient care for the encounter. The provider must manage the technology during the telehealth encounter and document the encounter in your EHR. The rules and regulations governing advanced nursing practice vary from state to state: full practice authority and restricted practice. In telehealth, rules and regulations include those from the origin site of services, the patient's location, and the provider's location.

LICENSURE AND CREDENTIALING

APNs are typically licensed in the state where they work. Telehealth patients may be located in another state, requiring the APRN to be licensed in every state where the patient is seen. There is a considerable variation in licensure and telehealth rules and regulations from state to state. (The APRN Consensus Model outlines roles and responsibilities for APRNs (https://www.ncsbn.org/public-files/aprn_consensus_model_by_state.pdf). Be familiar with the licensing and prescribing requirements when practicing telehealth. Another consideration is adhering to the Health Information Portability and Accountability Act of 1996 (HIPPA) providing privacy and security, Health Information Technology for Economic and Clinical Health (HITECH), and the Children's Online Privacy Protection Act (COPPA; Balestra, 2021). You should review the Centers for Medicare and Medicaid Services (CMS) fact sheet.

REIMBURSEMENT POLICIES

Reimbursement policies vary, based on state Medicaid and insurance plans. The Center for Medicare and Medicaid Services only reimburses for specific services using live video or they may designate specific areas, such as rural versus urban. During the

COVID-19 pandemic, Medicare waivers changed the reimbursement structure. CMS divides telehealth visits into three categories:

- **virtual visits:** a real-time clinical encounter using technology that supports real-time communication between clinician and patient
- **virtual check-ins:** a short patient-initiated action in which the clinician/patient already has a face-to-face or Virtual Visit and wants to check-in
- **eVisits:** a patient-initiated action in which the patient must initiate the initial inquiry or communication, often through a patient portal, and which can only be reported when the billing practice has an established relationship with the patient

You also will need to consider which patients are appropriate for virtual visits.

Questions to Consider When Using Telehealth

1. Which patients and diagnoses are easily handled virtually?
2. Which visits do we think must occur in person?
3. How often will we revisit these lists?
4. Does the home environment offer a space that is free from interruption?

Audio telehealth is a tool that can be used to reach patients in rural communities, individuals with disabilities, and others, providing a remote option that does not require broadband access. (U.S. Department of Health and Human Services [USDHHS], 2023). Audio-only telehealth is an effective way to reach vulnerable populations that can afford or do not have access to the required

TABLE 6.2 Summary of Medicare Services

Type of Service	What Is the Service?	HCPCS/CPT Code	Patient Relationship With Provider
Medicare Telehealth Visits	A visit with a provider that uses telecommunication systems between a provider and a patient	Common telehealth services include the following: • 99201–99215 (Office or other outpatient visits) • G0425–G0427 (Telehealth consultations, emergency department or initial inpatient) • G0406–G0408 (Follow-up inpatient telehealth consultations furnished to beneficiaries in hospitals or SNFs) For a complete list: https://www.cms.gov/Medicare/Medicare-General-Information/Telehealth/Telehealth-Codes	For new or established patients. To the extent the 1135 waiver requires an established relationship, HHS will not conduct audits to ensure that such a prior relationship existed for claims submitted during this public health emergency.
Virtual Check-In	A brief (5–10 minute) check-in with a practitioner via telephone or other telecommunications device to decide whether an office visit or other service is needed—a remote evaluation of recorded video and/or images submitted by an established patient	• HCPCS code G012 • HCPCS code G2010	For established patients
E-Visits	A communication between a patient and their provider through an online patient portal.	• 99421 • 99422 • 99423 • G2061 • G2062 • G2063	For established patients

Note. Adapted from Audio Only Telehealth, 2020.

video components. Many physicians use audio only, allowing them to provide equitable care. Communication technologies for audio-only telehealth may be found at https://www.hhs.gov/hipaa/for-professionals/privacy/guidance/hipaa-audio-telehealth/index.html.

CMS and many commercial payers modified payment policies in response to COVID-19 (Hollander & Carr, 2020):

- **permanent Medicare changes**
  - Federally Qualified Health Centers (FQHCs) and Rural Health Clinics (RHCs) can serve as distant site providers for behavioral/mental telehealth services.
  - Medicare patients can receive telehealth services for behavioral/mental health care in their homes.
  - No geographic restrictions exist for originating sites for behavioral/mental telehealth services.
  - Behavioral/mental telehealth services can be delivered using audio-only communication platforms.
  - Rural hospital emergency departments are accepted as originating sites.
- **temporary Medicare changes through December 31, 2024**
  - Federally Qualified Health Center (FQHC)/Rural Health Clinic (RHC) can be a distant site provider for non-behavioral/mental telehealth services.
  - Medicare patients can receive telehealth services authorized in their homes in the Calendar Year 2023 Medicare Physician Fee Schedule.
  - No geographic restrictions exist for originating sites for non behavioral/mental telehealth services.
  - Some non-behavioral/mental telehealth services can be delivered using audio-only communication platforms.

- An in-person visit within six months of an initial behavioral/mental telehealth service and annually after that is not required.
- Telehealth services can be provided by a physical therapist, occupational therapist, speech-language pathologist, or audiologist. (USDHHS, 2023)

REMAINING BARRIERS

- Reimbursement challenges top the list of physician-cited barriers to maintaining telehealth after COVID-19, followed by technology challenges for patients and liability concerns.
- Nearly two-thirds of physicians said lack of integration with EHRs would hinder their adoption of telehealth services.
- A total of 39.7% of consumers say their health system or insurance provider does not offer telehealth services, while another 34.6% said they are unaware if any service is offered (ATA, 2021).

ADDITIONAL RESOURCES

- telehealth in the time of COVID-19: https://www.cchpca.org/covid-19-actions/.
- coverage and benefits related to COVID-19 Medicaid and CHIP: https://www.cms.gov/files/document/03052020-medicaid-covid-19-fact-sheet.pdf.

CHAPTER SUMMARY

The pandemic telehealth response at the national, state, and local levels has been a significant step toward redesigning health care delivery (Kobiessi & Hickey, 2023). Telehealth has had a substantial impact on health care and has the potential to transform the way care is delivered (Doraiswamy et al., 2020). The rapid growth of telehealth during the pandemic led to an increased use of services. The weakness in our health care system that challenged and, in some cases, prevented the adoption of telehealth services has also been exacerbated (Curfman et al., 2021). Telehealth services offer convenience, cost savings, and increased access to care, but this innovation is not without its problems. More research is needed to identify the best practices in telehealth, and robust models of care must be created.

Food for Thought

1. What benefits do you see from the use of AI in the management of patients, and what are the downfalls?
2. Would you trust AI to help you make a clinical diagnosis?
3. What do you think is the best fit for telehealth?

KEY POINTS

- Telehealth can diagnose and treat acute and chronic illnesses and provide continuity of care over a distance.
- Providers must be familiar with the telehealth rules and regulations in their state and nationally.
- Health inequities still play a significant role in telehealth.

ACTIVITIES

1. Use the ATA's quick reference guide, "Quick Start Guide to Telehealth," to develop your sustainable telehealth company.
2. What areas and populations do you feel would be best served by telehealth?

REFERENCES

Association of American Medical Colleges [AAMC]. Telehealth competencies across the learning continuum. (2021). AAMC New and Emerging Areas in Medicine Series. https://store.aamc.org/downloadable/download/sample/sample_id/412/

Agency for Health care Research and Quality [AHRQ]. (2023). Project ECHO. Agency for Health Care Research and Quality. https://www.ahrq.gov/patient-safety/settings/multiple/project-echo/index.html

American Telehealth Association. (2023). *Telehealth: Defining 21st century care.* https://www.americantelemed.org/resource/why-telemedicine/

American Telehealth Association. (2021). *The adoption of telehealth.* https://www.americantelemed.org/resources/the-adoption-of-telehealth

American Telehealth Association. (2020). *Quick start guide to Telehealth during a health crisis.* https://cdn2.hubspot.net/hubfs/5096139/Files/Resources/ATA_QuickStart_Guide_to_Telehealth_4-10-20.pdf?__hstc=223170372.5a4e17347c27dfae5261ce606298cf4d.1680266172735.1680266172735.1680276123649.2&__hssc=223170372.3.1680276123649&__hsfp=3614612612&hsCtaTracking=f11af118-6144-4193-9a9e-7cc3773c2b8b%7C36ebfce7-8405-4789-959c-b1396226e32e

Balestra, M. (2018). Telehealth and legal implications for nurse practitioners. *The Journal for Nurse Practitioners, 14*(1), 33–39.

Board on Health Care Services, Institute of Medicine. (2012). *The role of telehealth in an evolving health care environment: Workshop summary.* National Academies Press (U.S.); Nov 20. 3, The Evolution of Telehealth: Where Have We Been and Where Are We Going? https://www.ncbi.nlm.nih.gov/books/NBK207141/

Centers for Medicare & Medicaid Services. (2020). *MEDICARE telemedicine health care provider fact sheet.* https://www.cms.gov/newsroom/fact-sheets/medicare-telemedicine-health-care-provider-fact-sheet

Curfman, A., McSwain, S. D., Chuo, J., Yeager-McSwain, B., Schinasi, D. A., Marcin, J., Herendeen, N., Chung, S. L., Rheuban, K., & Olson, C. A. (2021). Pediatric telehealth in the COVID-19 pandemic era and beyond. *Pediatrics, 148*(3), e2020047795. https://doi.org/10.1542/peds.2020-047795

DeNicola, N., Grossman, D., Marko, K., Sonalkar, S., Butler Tobah, Y. S., Ganju, N., Witkop, C. T., Henderson, J. T., Butler, J. L., & Lowery, C. (2020). Telehealth interventions to improve obstetric and gynecologic health outcomes: A systematic review. *Obstetrics and Gynecology, 135*(2), 371–382. https://doi.org/10.1097/AOG.0000000000003646

Doraiswamy, S., Abraham, A., Mamtani, R., & Cheema, S. (2020). Use of telehealth during the COVID-19 Pandemic: Scoping review. *J Med Internet Res., 22*(12):e24087. https://doi.org/10.2196/24087. PMID: 33147166; PMCID: PMC7710390.

Flodgren, G., Rachas, A., Farmer, A. J., Inzitari, M., & Shepperd, S. (2015). Interactive telemedicine: Effects on professional practice and health care outcomes. *The Cochrane Database of Systematic Reviews, 2015*(9), CD002098. https://doi.org/10.1002/14651858.CD002098.pub2

Hollander, J. E., & Carr, B. G. (2020). Virtually perfect? Telemedicine for COVID-19. *The New England Journal of Medicine, 382*(18), 1679–1681. https://doi.org/10.1056/NEJMp2003539

Institute of Medicine. (1996). *Telemedicine: A guide to assessing telecommunications for health care.* National Academy Press.

Kaplan, B. (2020). Revisiting health information technology ethical, legal and social issues and evaluation: Telehealth/telemedicine and COVID-19. *Int J Med Inform.*, 143, 104239. https://doi.org/10.1016/j.ijmedinf.2020.104239. PMID: 33152653; PMCID: PMC7831568

King-Dailey, K., Frazier, S., Bressler, S., & King-Wilson, J. (2022). The role of nurse practitioners in the management of heart failure patients and programs. *Current Cardiology Reports, 24*(12), 1945–1956. https://doi.org/10.1007/s11886-022-01796-0

Kobeissi, M. M., & Hickey, J. V. (2023). An infrastructure to provide safer, higher-quality, and more equitable telehealth. *Joint Commission Journal on Quality and Patient Safety, 49*(4), 213–222. https://doi.org/10.1016/j.jcjq.2023.01.006

Koonin, L. M., Hoots, B., Tsang, C. A., Leroy, Z., Farris, K., Tilman, J., Antall P., McCabe, B., Tong, I., & Harris, A. M. (2020). Trends in the use of telehealth during the emergence of the COVID-19 pandemic—United States, January–March 2020. *MMWR Morbidity and Mortality Weekly Report, 69*(43), 1595–1599. https://www.cdc.gov/mmwr/volumes/69/wr/mm6943a3.htm. PMID:33119561

Latifi, R., Doarn, C., & Merrell, R. C. (Eds.). (2021). *Telemedicine, telehealth and telepresence: Principles, strategies, applications, and new directions.* Springer. https://doi.org/10.1007/978-3-030-56917-4

Lee, H. S., & Kim, J. (2020). Development of a user needs-based telepresence robot for consultation. *Technology and Health Care: Official Journal of the European Society for Engineering and Medicine, 28*(1), 99–105. https://doi.org/10.3233/THC-191796

Mahtta, D., Daher, M., Lee, M. T., Sayani, S., Shishehbor, M., & Virani, S. S. (2021). Promise and perils of telehealth in the current era. *Current Cardiology Reports, 23*(9), 115. https://doi.org/10.1007/s11886-021-01544-w

Nesbitt, T. S. (2012), The evolution of telehealth: Where have we been and where are we going? Board on Health Care Services; Institute of Medicine. *The Role of Telehealth in an Evolving Health Care Environment: Workshop Summary.* National Academies Press (U.S.); 2012 Nov 20. 3 Washington, DC. https://www.ncbi.nlm.nih.gov/books/NBK207141/

National Organization of Nurse Practitioner Faculty [NONPF]. (2018). *NONPF supports telehealth in nurse practitioner education.* https://cdn.ymaws.com/www.nonpf.org/resource/resmgr/docs/telehealth_paper_final_20181.pdf

Nicosia, F. M., Kaul, B., Totten, A. M., Silvestrini, M. C., Williams, K., Whooley, M. A., & Sarmiento, K. F. (2021). Leveraging Telehealth to improve access to care: A qualitative evaluation of veterans' experience with the VA TeleSleep program. *BMC Health Services Research, 21*(1), 77. https://doi.org/10.1186/s12913-021-06080-5

Santomauro, C., McCurdie, T., Pollard, C., & Shuker, M. (2019). Exploring the feasibility of wearable technologies to provide interactive telepresence subspecialist support to remote clinicians treating patients with traumatic injuries. *Prehospital and Disaster Medicine, 34*(s1), s85–s85. https://doi.org/10.1017/S1049023X19001778

Snoswell, C. L., Taylor, M. L., Comans, T. A., Smith, A. C., Gray, L. C., & Caffery, L. J. (2020). Determining if telehealth can reduce health system costs: Scoping review. *Journal of Medical Internet Research, 22*(10), e17298. https://doi.org/10.2196/17298

U.S. Department of Health and Human Services [USDHHS]. (2023). Telehealth policy changes after the COVID-19 public health emergency. https://telehealth.hhs.gov/providers/policy-changes-during-the-covid-19-public-health-emergency/policy-changes-after-the-covid-19-public-health-emergency

U.S. Department of Health and Human Services [USDHHS]. (2023). Guidance on how the HIPAA rules permit covered health care providers and health plans to use remote communication technologies for audio-only telehealth. https://www.hhs.gov/hipaa/for-professionals/privacy/guidance/hipaa-audio-telehealth/index.html

Wijesooriya, N. R., Mishra, V., Brand, P. L. P., & Rubin, B. K. (2020). COVID-19 and telehealth, education, and research adaptations. *Paediatric Respiratory Reviews*, *35*, 38–42. https://doi.org/10.1016/j.prrv.2020.06.009

CHAPTER 7

APRNs in Leadership and Project Management

Linda Cole and Lisa Boss

OBJECTIVES

Upon completion of the chapter, the student will be able to

1. examine the role of APRNs in leadership
2. assess project management skills for APRNs
3. discuss the integration of leadership and project management in APRNs' practice

QUESTIONS/CHALLENGES

1. How can APRNs effectively lead interprofessional teams to improve patient care outcomes?
2. What are the essential project management skills that APRNs need to successfully plan, implement, and evaluate health care initiatives?

INTRODUCTION

In *The Future of Nursing: Leading Change, Advancing Health*, the Institute of Medicine (2011) noted that strong leadership is essential to transform health care and that all nurses must be leaders in the design, implementation, and evaluation of the health care system. Now, over 10 years later, that premise is still relevant. In Hamric's model of advanced practice nursing, defining characteristics of advanced practice registered nurses (APRNs) were identified, including primary criteria and core competencies, with leadership being one of those core competencies (Arslanian-Engoren, 2019). Leadership can be further stratified into clinical leadership, professional leadership, systems leadership, and health policy leadership (Carter & Reed, 2019). Clinical leadership occurs when APRNs build working relationships with health care team members, instill confidence in those they interact with, and problem-solve as part of the health care team (Carter & Reed, 2019). On the other hand, system leadership requires a big-picture view and a thorough understanding of the various components of health care delivery (Carter & Reed, 2019). Since APRNs are frequently considered frontline health care providers and, as such, are not recognized as formal leaders, since much of their time is spent in direct patient care (Lamb et al., 2018). APRNs must leverage clinical leadership and systems leadership skills to move health care delivery forward to improve patient care and the clinical practice of nurses and other health care professionals (Carter & Reed, 2019).

The COVID-19 pandemic demonstrated flaws in the health care system. In 2021 the American Association of Colleges of Nursing (AACN) released the *Essentials*, which outlines the expectation of APRNs to be trained to "apply quality improvement principles in care delivery and contribute to a culture of patient safety" (pp. 39–40) as well as "develop the capacity for leadership" (p. 54). APRNs must lead quality improvement initiatives which impact clinical care as well as health care systems.

Researchers noted that 70% of quality improvement (QI) initiatives fail, most within the first year (O'Donoghue et al., 2021). Quality improvement involves change, and change is hard to achieve. While clinicians often implement QI projects, they are frequently not involved in problem identification and solution development (O'Donoghue et al., 2021). APRNs are uniquely positioned to design and implement changes within the health care system. They have the opportunity to foster bidirectional leadership by using clinical and systems leadership skills to bring a problem to light without implying blame or having to solve it independently. To successfully lead change, APRNs must understand organizational culture and how to leverage influence.

ORGANIZATIONAL CULTURE

Organizational culture is based on three core components. The organization's values and vision form two components, while the assumptions and beliefs that leaders and staff members function under as each works in the organization comprise the third component (Thomas, 2023). Understanding organizational culture and readiness for change is key to successful leadership of quality initiatives (Thomas, 2022). Determining readiness for change can be done with various tools available (Table 7.1). Based on the organization's culture and readiness for change, the APRN can determine which aspect of the organization to focus their leadership efforts on.

Organizations can be broken into clinical microsystems, mesosystems, and macrosystems. A clinical "microsystem" is the smallest group of health care professionals working together regularly or intermittently to provide care to a discrete population of patients (Likosky, 2014). A clinical microsystem could be a single intensive care, medicine unit, or clinical section. Moving up the line, we have "mesosystems." These are described as linkages of clinical microsystems that allow them to move from disparate units to those supporting patients along their care continuum (Likosky, 2014). An example of a mesosystem

TABLE 7.1 Tools to Measure Readiness for Change

Focus	Tools
General Organizational Readiness	Dimensions of Organizational Readiness—Revised (DOOR-R) Organizational Readiness for Implementing Change (ORIC) Organizational Readiness to Change Assessment (ORCA) TCU Organizational Readiness for Change (TCU ORC)
Leadership Measures	Implementation Leadership Scale (ILS)
Culture and Climate Measures	Evidence-Based Practice Attitude Scale (EBPAS) Implementation Climate Scale (ICS) Organizational Culture Assessment Instrument (OCAI) Organizational Social Context (OSC) Measure
Program Fit Measures	Acceptability of Intervention Measure (AIM) Intervention Appropriateness Measure (IAM) Feasibility of Intervention Measure (FIM)
Other Measures	GEM-Dissemination and Implementation Initiative (GEM-D&I) Society for Implementation Research Collaboration (SIRC) Instrument Review Project

Note. Adapted from the California Evidence-Based Clearinghouse (CEBC).

could be the intensive care unit, the step-down unit, and the medical unit linked together to care for a particular patient population. Finally, the "macrosystem" is the unit that houses the microsystems and the mesosystem (Likosky, 2014). An example would be a hospital with multiple units caring for patient populations. When implementing change, it is important to identify which system will be affected and how a change in one could affect another. Strategies for implementing change and influence competencies may differ based on which system is impacted.

LEVERAGING INFLUENCE AND LEADING TEAMS

While APRNs are trained in clinical and systems leadership skills, they must realize they can influence others. Grenny and colleagues (2013) describe "influencers" as those who can create changes in human behavior. Influencers have a clear focus, use specific behaviors, and implement multiple types of influence, including personal, social, and structural approaches to achieve change (Gentry & Prince-Paul, 2021). By understanding influence, APRNs can influence change within organizations to implement quality initiatives, resulting in improved patient outcomes.

Another aspect of implementing change is working with teams. APRNs are involved in teams regularly as they care for patients. However, when implementing change, the APRN's role may shift from team member to team leader. One of the first steps in developing a team is to understand who the stakeholders are that the quality initiative will impact. It is essential to determine whether stakeholders will be part of the implementation team or simply kept informed regarding the progress of the quality initiative (Ogrinc et al., 2018). The team must then move from a group of individuals to a high-performance team that can implement the quality initiative.

To be an effective team leader, the APRN must employ specific approaches to succeed. One of those is adjusting the leadership style used to meet the team where it is at a particular stage of development (Wheelan et al., 2021). For example, in the early stages of team development, the leader may need to be more benevolent. As the team progresses, the leader may need to become more authoritative and then move into a facilitator role as the team matures. The team leader must be directive and confident as they facilitate open discussion of goals, tasks, and focus while providing feedback to the team (Wheelan et al., 2021). The team leader is responsible for holding team members accountable for the team's performance and providing guidance when needed. The team leader also has an opportunity to mentor team members in leadership by sharing the leadership functions of the team. The role of the team in quality initiative implementation is discussed further later in this chapter regarding project management.

CONCLUSION

APRNs have the knowledge and skills to expand their leadership potential from direct patient care to implementing changes that impact the clinical microsystems, mesosystems, and macrosystems. APRNs must clearly understand the needs of stakeholders while embracing leadership opportunities within health care teams. By expounding on these opportunities, APRNs can continue demonstrating their impact on positive patient and health care outcomes.

PROJECT MANAGEMENT

Lisa Boss, PhD, EdD, RN, CNS, CNE, CEN

What Is Project Management?

In health care, "project management" does not simply refer to managing a project. One of the most well-known definitions of project management (PM) defines it "as a temporary endeavor undertaken to produce a unique product, service, or result" (Project Management Institute [PMI], 2021, p. 245). In this definition, PM is a process that happens only one time and must include specific beginning and ending time points, a clearly defined scope, and specific outcome requirements that must be met (Heagney, 2022). Another definition of PM is "the application of knowledge, skills, tools, and techniques to project activities to meet the project requirements" (PMI, 2021, p. 245). From this perspective, a project may not necessarily occur only once but includes a specific process intended to meet a goal. While these two definitions are slightly different, they both assert that PM is a structured process intended to change the outcome of a problem (negative or positive).

Foundational PM Principles

Before attempting to lead or even develop a project, the APRN should be familiar with the "12 PM principles." Aligned with core values stated in the PMI Code of Ethics and Professional Conduct (2006), the 12 PM principles provide a foundational guideline for the project manager's strategy, decision-making, and problem-solving (PMI, 2021). These principles are not unique to the PM discipline; many overlap with traditional management principles used across many industries. As such, the APRN can interpret the 12 PM principles through a traditional management lens but, with advanced leadership skills, can also interpret the principles through a leadership lens specific to the health care setting.

The 12 PM principles are as follows (PMI, 2021, p. 23):

1. Be a diligent, respectful, and caring steward
2. Create a collaborative environment with stakeholders
3. Effectively engage with stakeholders
4. Focus on value
5. Recognize, evaluate, and respond to system interactions
6. Demonstrate leadership behaviors
7. Tailor based on context
8. Build quality into processes and deliverables
9. Optimize risk response
10. Embrace adaptability and resiliency
11. Enable change to achieve the envisioned future state

The American Nurses Association's (ANA) Code of Ethics (2015) is a well-known document containing "provisions" for a nurse to use when practicing in a manner consistent with quality nursing care and the ethical obligations of the profession. The essence of ANA's provisions is similar to PMI's (2021) 12 principles, providing the APRN with a solid foundation to guide their behaviors and actions throughout the PM process.

Performance Domains

Historically, the body of knowledge associated with PM was primarily focused on the *established process* or *steps* of managing a project. Whereas an established process was applicable to most projects in most industries and, if followed, was likely associated with success (PMI, 2021). In recent years, however, a paradigm shift in the PM industry reflects a clear change in focus. That is, the previous focus on the PM process was replaced with a focus on *teams* and *outcomes*. This drastic shift led to the creation of "performance domains," which guide PM behaviors and are considered essential for the effective delivery of project outcomes (PMI, 2021). The performance domains are stakeholders, team, development approach and life cycle, planning, project work, delivery, measurement, and uncertainty.

The eight performance domains are threads that run throughout a project. From the beginning to the end of a project, the performance domains are interconnected, and their influence can wax and wane, depending on the specific needs of the team and phase of the project. Different domains are more prominent during the project's various phases, allowing each project to be naturally tailored to its specific needs. For example, one project may have well-established relationships with stakeholders before the project's beginning, while another does not have well-established relationships with stakeholders. As a result, the team's performance related to developing working relationships with stakeholders will be different in the two projects.

TABLE 7.2 American Nurses Association Code of Ethics for Nurses

Provision 1	The nurse practices with compassion and respect for the inherent dignity, worth, and unique attributes of every person.
Provision 2	The nurse's primary commitment is to the patient, whether an individual, family, group, community, or population.
Provision 3	The nurse promotes, advocates for, and protects the rights, health, and safety of the patient.
Provision 4	The nurse has authority, accountability, and responsibility for nursing practice; makes decisions; and takes action consistent with the obligation to provide optimal patient care.
Provision 5	The nurse owes the same duties to self as to others, including the responsibility to promote health and safety, preserve wholeness of character and integrity, maintain competence, and continue personal and professional growth.
Provision 6	The nurse, through individual and collective effort, establishes, maintains, and improves the ethical environment of the work setting and conditions of employment that are conducive to safe, quality health care.
Provision 7	The nurse, in all roles and settings, advances the profession through research and scholarly inquiry, professional standards development, and the generation of both nursing and health policy.
Provision 8	The nurse collaborates with other health professionals and the public to protect human rights, promote health diplomacy, and reduce health disparities.
Provision 9	The profession of nursing, collectively through its professional organizations, must articulate nursing values, maintain the integrity of the profession, and integrate principles of social justice into nursing and health policy.

Note. *From American Nurses Association. (2015). Code of ethics with interpretative statements. Silver Spring, MD: Author. Retrieved from http://www.nursingworld.org/MainMenuCategories/EthicsStandards/CodeofEthicsforNurses/Code-ofEthics-For-Nurses.html.*

STAKEHOLDER PERFORMANCE

Developing a productive working relationship with stakeholders throughout the project's duration is key in the stakeholder performance domain. Stakeholders who support project outcomes are satisfied, whereas stakeholders who oppose the project or outcomes could negatively impact all project phases (PMI, 2021). To gain support from stakeholders, clear and frequent communication is necessary. In addition, the APRN must astutely understand stakeholders' perspectives to adjust their behavior for this domain effectively. The APRN should analyze each stakeholder according to power, expectations, degree of influence, and interest in the project to ensure collaboration in managing expectations, negotiation, problem-solving, and decision-making is as seamless as possible (PMI, 2021).

TEAM PERFORMANCE

To achieve a high-performing team, specific aspects related to the activities and functions of all team members, team culture, and the environment are necessary to foster team cohesiveness, shared leadership, and leadership behaviors from all team members (PMI, 2021). The APRN is responsible for establishing a clear vision and objectives, roles and responsibilities of team members, effective team communication, and guidance to keep the project moving forward. In addition, identifying areas where the team performs well and those where it could improve performance is necessary. To establish a safe, respectful, nonjudgmental environment, desired behaviors for the APRN include transparency, integrity, respect, positive discourse, support, courage, and celebrating success. On the other hand, conflict management skills are necessary and include keeping communication open and respectful, focusing on issues and not people, focusing on the present and future without dwelling in the past, and searching for resolutions or alternatives together as a team (PMI, 2021).

DEVELOPMENT APPROACH AND LIFE CYCLE PERFORMANCE

This domain focuses on activities associated with the development approach, cadence, and project life cycle phases (PMI, 2021). The development approach refers to how the project or product is created and evolves throughout the project's life cycle. The APRN should be knowledgeable about different development approaches to ensure the most appropriate approach fits with the nature of the project. For example, a predictive approach is useful when essential details of the project are defined, collected, and analyzed at the start of a project. On the other hand, an adaptive approach is most useful when program requirements are likely to change throughout the project process due to uncertainty or volatility. "Cadence" refers to the timing and frequency of project deliverables; the APRN must determine whether there is a single, multiple, periodic, or continuous delivery approach to keep the project's momentum on track and moving forward. The life cycle and number of phases for a project vary greatly and are interconnected to the chosen development approach and cadence. Examples of different phases in a life cycle of a project can include feasibility, design, build, test, deploy, and close (PMI, 2021). The primary role of the APRN in this domain is to align best the development approach, cadence, and life cycles to easily address threats to the project, as well as eliminate uncertainty among team members.

PLANNING PERFORMANCE

The purpose of the planning domain is for the PM to proactively develop an approach to create the project deliverables and outcomes (PMI, 2021). The APRN will drive the amount of planning throughout the project's life cycle. Awareness of the amount, timing, and frequency is important because every project is unique and can be influenced by the development approach, nature of deliverables, organizational requirements and policies and procedures, market conditions directly or indirectly affecting the budget, and legal and regulatory processes. The APRN will need to accurately estimate work effort for the team and others, costs, physical resources, and duration of the project. Developing an accurate schedule for the project will serve as a blueprint to keep the team on track. Effective communication, one of the key advanced leadership skills for the APRN, is perhaps the most important skill to effectively guide the project's work and deliver outcomes (PMI, 2021).

PROJECT WORK PERFORMANCE

The project work performance domain refers to establishing the specific processes and executing the work that will allow the team to deliver expected deliverables and outcomes (PMI, 2021). The most important foci for the APRN in this domain are managing workflow, keeping the team focused, establishing efficient processes, managing supplies and logistics, working with outside contractors and vendors, monitoring and adapting to project plan changes, and communicating effectively. Another key leadership skill for the APRN is to acknowledge and manage lessons learned and actively strategize to improve anticipated challenges in the project based on the lessons learned. Continuous learning and making process adjustments throughout the project will lead to more efficient project performance, effective physical and financial resources management, and overall process improvement (PMI, 2021).

DELIVERY PERFORMANCE

In this domain, the goal for the APRN is to focus on meeting requirements, scope, and quality expectations that produce the anticipated deliverables that drive project outcomes (PMI, 2021). In the context of PM, requirements are conditions or capabilities that must be present in a product, service, or result to satisfy a business need (PMI, 2021). The APRN should actively elicit requirements at the beginning of a project, be flexible when new requirements evolve or are discovered throughout the project, and effectively manage requirements so that the project remains on track. Regardless of when a requirement is identified, stakeholder support is critical for project success (PMI, 2021). The scope is another important element in this domain and is directly related to the identified requirements. Scope represents the sum of products, services, and results that need to be provided for a successful project. The APRN has a valuable role in clearly defining the scope of a project so that the requirements developed result in a successful project as well as stakeholder support (PMI, 2021). Aside from the scope and requirements for a project, quality is an important element in this domain. Quality is the degree to which a set of inherent project characteristics fulfill requirements (PMI, 2021). Thus, the APRN's role in quality is to balance the needs of the project's processes and products with the cost of meeting those needs. PM components relevant to this category include costs associated with overhead, training, and process audits of the project (PMI, 2021).

MEASUREMENT PERFORMANCE

The measurement performance domain involves assessing project performance and having appropriate methods in place to intervene using baseline data to maintain optimal performance (PMI, 2021). The APRN must employ effective measures that accurately track, evaluate, and report data that communicates project statuses to team members and stakeholders. Leading and lagging indicators are the most common quantifiable measures used to evaluate performance. Together, effective use of leading and lagging indicators predict changes and trends in the project and reveal past performance or conditions that are directly related to the project outcomes and/or deliverables (PMI, 2021). The APRN must choose specific, meaningful, achievable, relevant, and timely metrics to accurately measure a specific data point. Common data points amenable to measurement include baseline performance, resources, business value, stakeholder satisfaction, and forecasts (PMI, 2021). The use of dashboards, visual charts (pie and stop-light), and big visible charts are helpful to convey data points easily to team members and stakeholders so that the information is accurately represented (PMI, 2021). Finally, the APRN must actively identify measurement pitfalls, including the Hawthorne effect, confirmation bias, and an accurate understanding of correlation versus causation. When data points such as schedule and budget are outside of predicted ranges, the APRN must effectively trouble-shoot performance so that the project team can take immediate action to identify the variance (PMI, 2021).

UNCERTAINTY PERFORMANCE

This final domain refers to the uncertainty related to any project. Uncertainty is a state of not knowing or unpredictability, which is inherent in every project (PMI, 2021). Different types of uncertainty include ambiguity, complexity, volatility, and overall project risk. Recognizing and responding to uncertainty is crucial for the APRN to navigate all types of uncertainty effectively. Strategies for proactively responding to uncertainty include gathering information, preparing for multiple outcomes, and building a team culture of resilience (PMI, 2021). In addition, the APRN must be skilled in anticipating and responding to threats that potentially have a negative impact on the project. Strategies to deal with threats differ in every project, including avoidance, escalation, transferring ownership, mitigation, and acceptance (PMI, 2021). One way to proactively prevent threats is the APRN's awareness of opportunities that improve project performance and/or outcomes. With established mechanisms to identify threats and leverage opportunities, the APRN can guide the team to maintain alignment with established project outcomes (PMI, 2021).

TABLE 7.3 The Project Management Institute's Eight Performance Domains

Domain	Focus
Stakeholder Performance	To address activities and functions associated with stakeholders (p. 8).
Team Performance	To address activities and functions associated with the people who are responsible for producing project deliverables that realize business outcomes (p. 16).
Development Approach and Life Cycle Performance	To address activities and functions associated with the development approach, cadence, and life cycle phases of the project (p. 32).
Planning Performance	To address activities and functions associated with the initial, ongoing, and evolving organization and coordination necessary for delivering project deliverables and outcomes (p. 51).
Project Work Performance	To address activities and functions associated with establishing project processes, managing physical resources, and fostering a learning environment (p. 69).
Delivery Performance	To address activities and functions associated with delivering the scope and quality that the project was undertaken to achieve (p. 81).
Measurement Performance	To address activities and functions associated with assessing project performance and taking appropriate actions to maintain acceptable performance (p. 93).
Uncertainty Performance	To address activities and functions associated with risk and uncertainty (p. 116).

Note. From *Project Management Institute*, 2021.

Conclusion

A recent paradigm shift in the PM industry reflects a focus on teams and outcomes rather than simply guiding a team through the PM process. With advanced leadership skills, the APRN is positioned to build relationships with interdisciplinary team members effectively, oversee each step in the PM process, and lead the team to meet or exceed established project outcomes in a complex and rapidly changing health care environment. Using the eight performance domains outlined by the Project Management Institute (2021) and advanced leadership skills, the APRN's role in PM is clearly defined, and successfully leading an interdisciplinary team through a project is a realistic expectation.

CHAPTER SUMMARY

As clinical leaders, APRNs easily build working relationships and lead interdisciplinary teams to accomplish excellent patient outcomes. APRNs can expand their expertise from clinical patient care to include robust leadership skills that will directly impact our flawed health care system in meaningful and relevant ways. By acquiring and applying elements of systems leadership skills, such as quality improvement and project management, APRNs can have a profound effect on change at the microsystems, mesosystems, and macrosystems levels, ultimately positively impacting patient and health care outcomes.

Food for Thought

How would you approach project leadership? What are your leadership skills?

KEY POINTS

- APRNs must leverage clinical and system leadership skills to improve patient outcomes and health care delivery.
- Understanding organizational culture and readiness for change is key to a successful implementation of quality initiatives.
- In health care, "PM" does not simply refer to managing a project. PM is a structured process intended to change the outcome of a problem (negative or positive).
- The APRN should know the 12 PM principles (PMI, 2021) before beginning the PM process.
- The PM process is guided by eight performance domains: stakeholder, team, life cycle, planning, project work, delivery, measurement, and uncertainty.
- Equipped with advanced leadership skills and guided by the PM process, the APRN is positioned to lead an interdisciplinary team systematically and successfully through the PM process.

ACTIVITIES

Discussion Board Questions or Personal Reflection Questions

1. How would you describe your ability to influence others and lead quality initiatives?
2. Reflect on a past or current practice setting and think of a problem that would lend itself well to the PM process. In the context of the PM performance domains, how would you begin to determine the appropriate stakeholders to address the problem and develop a productive working relationship?
3. Considering the previous question, how would you develop a high-performing team? How would you define or determine if your team is "high performing"?

Course Paper Suggestion

1. Faculty could have students develop a paper on high-performing teams and what characteristics those teams might possess.
2. Faculty could assign a course paper that requires students to identify a past or current problem in the practice setting and describe how they would address the problem in the context of the PM domains outlined in the PMBOK guide (2021). Depending on the course requirements, the level of detail in each performance domain could vary as the faculty deems appropriate.

REFERENCES

American Association of Colleges on Nursing. (2021). *The essentials: Core competencies for professional nursing education.* https://www.aacnnursing.org/Portals/42/AcademicNursing/pdf/Essentials-2021.pdf

American Nurses Association. (2015). *Code of ethics with interpretive statements.* Silver Spring. http://www.nursingworld.org/MainMenuCategories/EthicsStandards/CodeofEthicsforNurses/Code-ofEthics-For-Nurses.html

Arslanian-Engoren, C. (2019). Conceptualizations of advanced practice nursing. In M.F. Tracy & E.T. O'Grady (Eds.), *Hamric and Hanson's advanced practice nursing: An integrative approach* (6th ed., 25–60). Elsevier.

California Evidence-Based Clearinghouse. (2023). *Implementation measures.* https://www.cebc4cw.org/implementing-programs/tools/measures/

Carter, M., & Reed, L. (2019). Leadership. In M. F. Tracy, & E. T. O'Grady (Eds.), *Hamric and Hanson's advanced practice nursing: An integrative approach* (6th ed., 256–285). Elsevier.

Gentry, H., & Prince-Paul, M. (2021). The nurse influencer: A concept synthesis and analysis. *Nursing Forum, 56*(1), 181–187. https://doi.org/10.1111/nuf.12516

Grenny, J., Patterson, K., Maxfield, D., McMillan, R., & Switzler, A. (2013). *Influencer: The new science of leading change* (2nd ed.). McGraw Hill.

Heagney, J. (2022). *Fundamentals of project management* (6th ed.). Harper Collins Leadership.

Institute of Medicine. (2011). *The Future of nursing: Leading change, advancing health.* National Academies Press.

Kalmakis, K. (2021). Beyond the discipline: Nurse practitioner members and leaders of interdisciplinary research teams. *Journal of the American Association of Nurse Practitioners, 33*(5), 405–408. https://doi.org/10.1097/JXX.0000000000000376

Lamb, A., Martin-Misener, R., Bryant-Lukosius, D., & Latimer, M. (2018). Describing the leadership capabilities of advanced practice nurses using a qualitative study. *Nursing Open, 5*(3) 400–413. https://doi.org/10.1002/nop2.150

Likosky, D. S. (2014). Clinical microsystems: A critical framework for crossing the quality chasm. *Journal of ExtraCorpeal Technology, 46*(1), 33–37.

O'Donoghue, S. C., DiLibero, J., & Altman, M. (2021). Leading sustainable quality improvement. *Nursing Management, 52*(2), 42–50. https://doi.org/10.1097/01.NUMA.0000724940.43792.86

Ogrinc, G. S., Headrick, L. A., Barton, A. J., Dolansky, M. A., Madigosky, W. S., & Miltner, R. S. (2018). Appendix: Tools to help your improvement. In Authors (Eds.) *Fundamentals of health care improvement: A guide to improving your patients' care* (3rd ed., pp. 159–180). Joint Commission Resources & Institute for Health Care Improvement.

Project Management Institute. (2006). *Code of ethics and professional conduct.* Project Management Institute. https://www.pmi.org/-/media/pmi/documents/public/pdf/ethics/pmi-code-of-ethics.pdf?rev=6af21906e5934b638ceeabeb4137f41d&la=en

Project Management Institute. (2021). *The standard for project management and a guide to the management body of knowledge* (PMBOK guide; 7th ed.). Project Management Institute.

Thomas, L. W. (2022). Quality improvement: Assessing your clinical microsystem. *Nephrology Nursing Journal, 49*(2). 103–107.

Thomas, P. L. (2023). Beyond plans: Strategic practices in achieving organizational effectiveness. In L. A. Roussel, P. L. Thomas, & J. A. Harris (Eds.), *Management and leadership for nurse administrators* (9th ed., pp. 113–130). Jones & Bartlett Learning.

Wheelan, S. A., Akerlund, M., & Jacobsson, C. (2021). Effective team leadership. In Authors (Eds.) *Creating effective teams: A guide for members and leaders* (6th ed., pp. 65–82). Sage Publishing.

CHAPTER 8

Health Policy and Advocacy

What Can Advanced Practice Nurses Do?

Kathleen Siders, Robert Carl Coghlan III, and Aastha Krebs

OBJECTIVES

Upon completion of the chapter, the student will be able to

1. describe how health policy impacts practice
2. discuss the complex role organizations play in the profession and society
3. analyze relevant internal and external factors that drive health care costs and reimbursement

QUESTIONS/CHALLENGES

1. How would you advocate for advanced practice nurses?
2. How would you advocate for an underserved population?

INTRODUCTION

The health care sector represents a large part of the economy of the United States. The Centers for Medicare and Medicaid Services (CMS) estimated that in 2021, the United States spent approximately $4.31 trillion, or 18.3% of the gross domestic product reflecting strong growth in Medicaid and private health insurance

(CMS, 2023). As health care becomes more complex, both in technology and in regard to the personnel who care for patients, costs will continue to rise. Nurses are in a key position to help guide health policy in the future. Nursing is at the heart of all aspects of patient care. Advanced practice registered nurses (APRNs) are uniquely positioned to provide care from the bedside to the boardroom. APRNs serve as administrators, clinicians, and educators. They hold positions of influence throughout organizations that seek to influence policy at all levels of government, from the local arena to the federal and even international level. APRNs must accept, embrace, and protect this position of power.

POLICY DEFINITIONS

The study of policy is both an art and a science. Nursing is an art requiring thought and finesse in development and science using quantitative and qualitative methods to express and develop policy. "Policy" is defined as a means or set of actions to set a direction for a specific topic (Motacki & Burke, 2017). For example, public policy establishes goals or actions to influence the process. Public policy defines a concern or position that society is to follow. This is not limited to governmental entities but also involves health care, industries, educational institutions, private groups, and other organizations. A policy is a perspective or action sought by the group in question. "Health policy" is a set of goals or actions that seek to establish a specific plan to create a wholesale change or adjust the current process. This could be something like the development of Medicare and Medicaid in 1965 or the Affordable Care Act of the 21st century. Health policy includes laws passed by legislative bodies and subsequent rules that affect patient care and care delivery.

Nurses must understand the development and implications of policy. As a group, nurses must be on the ground floor of legal developments impacting licensure and ability to care for our patients. Ideally, policies are designed to elaborate on what is wanted and how to best get there.

POLICY CHANGE

The best way to achieve change is at the grassroots level. Advocacy is a process whereby an individual or a group seeks to influence a specific political process or the allocation of resources. Nursing already has a process in place to advocate for change. We need to identify the exact problem cause(s) and define the problem in easily understood terms. Once defined, nurses must identify potential solutions as well as outline their costs. Costs may seem foreign to nurses, and they are not exclusively financial. For example, there may be implementation costs associated with a given solution, such as determining whether additional nurses will need to be hired, how many are required, what specialty or level of experience will be needed, and whether there will be adequate college- or university-level resources to provide additional education. The fiscal impact also includes the patient and system's cost savings.

Another point to consider is the impact of the policy on the system in general. Will access to care improve? Will system stability improve? Finally, what is the target objective to be achieved? The answers to these questions should be clearly stated so that anyone involved in the process can better understand the goal. One aspect often overlooked in policy is the evaluation phase. The process and outcomes must periodically be re-evaluated whether the policy is totally, partially, or not implemented. If partially implemented, what were the key elements, and why? If not implemented, what can be retooled and presented again?

An illustrative example is the Clinton Health Care Initiative of the early 1990s. Although Congress did not implement the plan, key plan elements were subsequently used, namely the Health Insurance Portability and Accountability Act (HIPAA) and the

Children's Health Insurance Program (CHIP). Most of Congress supported the policy initiatives, and President Clinton signed the programs into law. Another example was the Emergency Medical Treatment and Labor Act (EMTALA) as part of the Consolidated Omnibus Budget Reconciliation Act (COBRA) in 1987. These examples show how bipartisanship often leads to the most effective policy initiatives.

HOW POLICY IMPACTS HEALTH CARE

Policy impacts health care and represents an integral part of the health care system by directly shaping the public's health and well-being. Policies set at the local, state, or national level impact issues upon which the entire health care system is based, such as access, coverage, costs, delivery, and privacy. Additionally, several health care policies such as patient care, employee health care policies, drug policies, and security and privacy policies establish guidelines for the health care system to benefit nurses. This also impacts other issues adjacent yet relevant to health care, such as public health campaigns and social barriers to health care access based on income, inclusivity, and minority community access (Rogers, 2022).

The Affordable Care Act of March 2010 reformed the U.S. health care system and focused on decreasing the number of people without health insurance. Before the law's passage, 15% of the U.S. population was uninsured. By 2018, the uninsured rate declined to 8.5%, resulting in 18 million more people with health insurance coverage (Antos & Capretta, 2020). The nonelderly uninsured rate declined from 17.8% in 2010 to 10.2% in 2021, driven by Medicaid and non-group coverage increases. Provisions in the Families First Coronavirus Act also prohibited states from disenrolling people from Medicaid until after the COVID-19 public health emergency. The American Rescue Plan Act also provided enhanced Affordable Care Act marketplace subsidies (Tolbert et al., 2022).

Surprise medical billing was an important health care cost issue solved via policy. Before the No Surprises Act, patients could be billed for receiving care from an out-of-network provider or out-of-network facility, even unknowingly or if their plan did not cover the entire out-of-network cost. As of February 2020, 41% of insured adults in the United States had a surprise medical bill within the past 2 years, 19% due to receiving care from an out-of-network provider. Out-of-network charges could also result from being treated by an out-of-network physician, riding in an out-of-network ambulance, or being taken to an out-of-network hospital in an emergency. Notably, 18% of emergency department visits resulted in at least one surprise medical bill (Pollitz et al., 2022). The No Surprises Act became federal law in January 2022 and featured several protections to eliminate surprise medical billing for most emergency services as well as out-of-network cost sharing for most emergency and some nonemergency services. The law also covered anesthesiology or radiology services provided at the patient's in-network facility and required health care providers and facilities to provide patients easy-to-understand explanations of billing protections (CMS, 2022b). The Health Insurance Portability and Accountability Act (HIPAA) requires medical providers to adhere to federal and state data privacy laws to protect patient information, including the Fair Credit Reporting Act, the Gramm-Leach-Bliley Act, and the Family Educational Rights and Privacy Act. Additionally, in 2022, the American Data Privacy and Protection Act (ADPPA) was introduced to Congress, to update HIPAA and data privacy legislation. The ADPPA allows consumers to opt out of targeted advertisements, protects consumer data privacy and data protection safeguards, and regulates health data apps that host data unregulated by HIPPA and not currently covered by the law (McKeon, 2022).

HIPAA became law in August 1996 and represented a policy effort to codify patients' medical information privacy. One of the law's aims was to "improve the portability and accountability of health insurance coverage" and prevent waste, fraud, and abuse in the health care sector (The HIPAA Guide, 2017). Significantly, the law mandated a set of privacy and security rules for "protected health information," to which the Department of Health and Human Services required compliance in April 2003. This protected information was defined as "any information held by a covered entity which concerns health status, the provision of health care, or payment for health care that can be linked to an individual" (The HIPAA Journal, 2023). The HIPAA Security Rule updated the law to account for the electronic storage of information and became effective in April 2005. HIPAA was updated again to account for changes in the digital storage of information and the occurrence of data breaches, which led to the HIPAA Breach Notification Rule in September 2009, and then the Omnibus Final Rule became effective in March 2013 replacing a controversial "risk of harm" breach standard from an earlier version of the rule. Despite implementing these rules to secure patient data, many entities failed to comply fully with the law. The policy response was the HIPAA Enforcement Rule, passed in March 2006, which allowed HHS to investigate rule violations and breaches. The Health Information Technology for Economic and Clinical Health Act, passed in 2009, was a policy initiative to encourage health care providers to adopt electronic records and introduced the meaningful use. Meaningful Use is an electronic health record incentive program run by the CMS. providing a financial incentive for the use of HER technology to achieve health and efficiency goals.

Child immunization is a critical case study of policy's substantial impact on health care. As late as the 1990s, nearly half of the children in the United States lacked immunizations at the proper times. The Clinton administration set a key health care policy objective for all children to receive immunizations by age 3. Due to strong evidence-based policy showing universal immunization benefits public health, an influential organizational movement promoted the effort, increasing children's immunization to 90%. Promoters of the policy onboarded states, professional organizations, health care professionals, and funding from Congress to subsidize immunizations. They also applied systems used to track animal immunizations to children. Measures were implemented to ensure compliance, including denying enrollment in Head Start and child centers and withholding benefits from the Special Supplemental Program for Women, Infants, and Children (Institute of Medicine, 2008).

Policies restricting tobacco sales also demonstrate a substantial impact on health care. The Trump administration banned some flavored e-cigarettes in January 2020 to reduce the increasing teenage use of vaping products (Kirkham, 2020). Before the ban, the Federal Drug Administration (FDA) issued over 8,600 warning letters and 1,000 civil monetary penalties to retailers. In collaboration with the Federal Trade Commission (FTC), the FDA banned e-liquid products that resembled child-friendly products. "The Real Cost" youth e-cigarette prevention campaign was launched targeting teenagers via television, digital, and social media advertising (FDA, 2019). Teen e-cigarette usage rose from 1.5% to 27.5% between 2011 and 2019, despite teen cigarette usage declining from 15.8% to 5.8% during the same period. Following the ban, 14.1% of high school students and 3.3% of middle school students reported current e-cigarette use in 2021, a substantial decline (FDA, 2019). Earlier policies targeting general tobacco use were also effective in reducing smoking rates. Consumption taxes reduced usage at a price elasticity rate of –0.37%, or a 3.7% reduction per 10% tax increase. Smoke-free air laws banning smoking in indoor public spaces were also effective at reducing tobacco use, with a 10% relative reduction at 25% initial smoking prevalence, reducing youth cigarette use by 15%. Other measures also reduced tobacco consumption, such as a 10% to 15% reduction attributed to comprehensive tobacco control programs in the U.S., a 20% to 25% drop due to mass anti-tobacco public health campaigns, and a 12% to 20% drop due to health warnings. Additionally, marketing bans resulted in a 12% drop in European countries between 1990 to 2005 (Levy et al., 2018).

Rural health care also presents a significant set of issues and challenges for policy implementation. Rural Americans typically face higher uninsured rates and limited access to nearby hospitals. However, Medicaid expansion has increased the number of open hospitals and increased the insured rates by an average of 16% in 36 states that implemented the program, including Montana, New Mexico, and Arizona (Hoadley et al., 2018; National Conference of State Legislators [NCSL], 2020). The ACA also improved health care by lowering the rate of rural Americans without health insurance and increasing the number of insurers in the ACA marketplace, creating more health insurance coverage options for rural Americans. Rural areas typically face the challenge of closing hospitals. Policy responses included Tennessee's 2018 Rural Hospital Transformation Act, which directed the Tennessee Department of Economic and Community Development to establish "transformation plans" for rural hospitals, including measures to improve the hospital's business model. Alabama, Georgia, and Vermont passed similar legislation to prevent rural hospital closures. Additionally, the policy encourages the adoption of alternative payment models for paying rural hospitals and moving away from fee-for-service payments to keep the hospital open. Several states, including Pennsylvania, Oregon, and Texas, are pursuing alternatives. Pennsylvania developed the Pennsylvania Rural Health Model, which allocated global budgets for participating hospitals and established the Rural Health Redesign Center in 2019 to provide technical assistance to 13 participating hospitals (NCSL, 2020).

To comply with the Supremacy Clause of the U.S. Constitution, local-level policies created by a lower level of government must comply with those created by a higher level (e.g., federal or state; Constitution of the United States, 1787). "Ceiling preemption" is a process whereby the higher level of government may prevent a local-level policy from being enacted and enforced (Rutkow et al., 2008). While doing so may limit innovative policies at the lower level, public policy can be rapidly created, enacted, and enforced by other means, such as judicial opinions and presidential and gubernatorial executive orders (American Bar Association, 2021). Under the preemptive doctrine, state governments can annul local laws inconsistent with state laws. During the COVID-19 pandemic, polarized political issues, such as COVID-19 restrictions, were prime examples of state preemption. In 2020, Arizona Governor Douglas A. Ducey issued a gubernatorial executive order to bar the local government from "restricting persons from leaving their home due to the COVID-19 public health emergency" (Ducey, 2020). Governor Ducey's executive order prevented city and county governments from imposing COVID-19 restrictions stricter than the state was willing to impose and enforce. Similar state preemptions were enforced in Florida, Texas, Tennessee, Mississippi, and West Virginia, among others, leading to stifled local emergency response to the pandemic. The effects of housing insecurity, lack of access to internet-assisted health care, and paid sick leave disproportionately affected low-wage workers, minorities, and women.

In Cedar Rapids, Iowa, Mayor Brad Hart sought to exercise special mayoral powers given during the emergency state to implement city-level stay-at-home orders. However, in April 2020, Iowa Governor Kim Reynolds and the Iowa attorney general opposed such orders restricting public movement, citing that city, county, and other local-level governments do not have the authority to impose and enforce business closures, mask mandates, or stay-at-home orders (Mervosh & Healy, 2020). Iowa did not have a statewide order at the time, and with Governor Reynolds's preemption, Mayor Hart could not issue city ordinances to limit the spread of COVID-19. However, Mayor Hart creatively curtailed the preemption by restricting public access to or shutting down public buildings, libraries, public transit systems, parks, and playgrounds. In the following months, COVID-19 cases in Iowa surged to more than 4,100 people testing positive for the virus daily. In mid-November 2020, amidst growing pressure from the public, city mayors, health care professionals, and the Iowa State Board of Health, Governor Reynolds reversed her stance, issuing a limited mask mandate and social isolation precautions (Mervosh et al., 2020).

ADVOCATING FOR CHANGE

A commonly asked, yet pressing, question is how a nurse can effect change in the complex health care policy arena. There is a saying in political science that all politics are local. This means that any political process starts and ends at the local level. The most basic level is to be active in your local nursing organization. The local organization receives updates from state and national organizations and is a conduit for the information flow. They also provide an opportunity for members at the local level to study and review information to decide their position of support. Another consideration is serving on committees at all levels of organizations. The main work of any organization occurs in its committees. The decisions or planning that takes place there influences the direction of policies that will potentially influence the national organization's decisions. There are also opportunities to participate in committee leadership roles to help shape the direction of policies. These roles also allow nurses to advocate for change across the policy spectrum.

APRNs utilize research to substantiate their positions on varying different policy perspectives. Many aspects of these politics are driven by emotion. However, for them to be long-standing and long-lasting policy changes, decision-makers must be driven by facts. APN is well grounded in theory and how to design research to answer specific questions. Part of this includes consuming, critically evaluating, and reviewing published research. Does the research present adequately answer the question posed?

ACCESS TO HEALTH CARE

Policies directly shape the health of a nation. Healthy People 2030 has several objectives related to health care access, such as the availability of preventative services, reducing wait times at emergency departments, availability of prenatal and perinatal care, and providing access to dental insurance and care. Access to health care is a significant issue in the United States, with 16.6% of the nonelderly (less than 65 years old) population lacking health insurance in 2013, before the enactment of the Affordable Care Act (ACA, 2010; Altman, 2016). Among 11 developed high income countries—Australia, Canada, France, Germany, the Netherlands, New Zealand, Norway, Sweden, Switzerland, the United Kingdom, and the United States—the United States has continuously ranked at the bottom of this metric since 2004 (Schneider et al., 2021). Analysis of performance measures across five domains—access to care, care process, administrative efficiency, equity, and health care outcomes—included 71 performance metrics. In the 2021 report, the United States was an outlier, with significantly lower scores in all domains except the care process, ranking 2nd in that domain and 11th in all others. Norway, the Netherlands, and Australia ranked as the three top-performing countries.

The 2012 National Health Care Disparities Report indicated that while health care quality in the United States is improving, it remains subpar for minorities and low-income individuals.

Additionally, the report indicated that access to health care was worsening, especially related to health care access disparities based on race and income level (Agency for Health Care Research and Quality, 2013). These racial and income-based health disparities, especially in infant mortality rates and average life expectancy, may be responsible for poor health indicators in the United States compared to other industrialized countries (Central Intelligence Agency [CIA], 2022a; CIA, 2022b).

The establishment of the Medicare and Medicaid programs in 1965 and the ACA in 2010 are inarguably the most impactful health-related legislation in the United States. In the landmark amendment of the Public Health Service Act of 1944 (PHSA; Public Law 78-410), the Patient Protection and Affordable Care Act (PPACA; Public Law 111–148) was enacted by the 111th U.S. Congress and signed into law by President Barack Obama in 2010. The provisions of the ACA went into effect between 2014 and 2020 in a phased manner. In June 2009, President Barack Obama stated at the Annual Conference of the American Medical Association,

> The cost of our health care is a threat to our economy. It is an escalating burden on our families and businesses. It is a ticking time bomb for the federal budget and is unsustainable for the United States of America ... health care is the most important thing we can do for America's long-term fiscal health. That is a fact. (White House, 2009)

This excerpt from Obama's speech succinctly addresses the need for ACA.

The ACA significantly reformed the health sector by expanding health insurance access to 32 million previously uninsured and significantly aided older adults, low-income individuals, and minority groups. Costing an estimated $1.8 trillion between 2012 and 2022, the ACA sourced funding from various new taxes, health plan fees, individual and employer insurance mandates, and cost containment efforts in Medicare and Medicaid programs. Some of the ACA's most noteworthy provisions include banning denial of coverage due to preexisting conditions, eliminating lifetime limitations for treating illnesses, free preventative care, eliminating or restricting lifetime coverage or annual limits, prohibiting or rescinding coverage except for fraud, and mandating access to out of network emergency care.

The major goals of the ACA were the following:

1. To expand health insurance coverage for the people in the United States.
2. To expand Medicaid to cover all adults with income below 138% of the federal poverty level (FPL).
3. To support innovative medical care delivery methods designed to lower health care costs generally. (U.S. Department of Health and Human Services [HHS], 2022a)

Some important provisions of the ACA to meet these goals include providing households with incomes between 100% and 400% of the FPL with premium tax credits to lower the cost of health insurance; eliminating insurance coverage denial based on preexisting conditions; eliminating dollar or days and lifetime or annual limitations on the treatment of illnesses; allowing individuals up to age 26 to remain on their parent's insurance plans, regardless of factors like marital status, financial independence, and living arrangements; and free preventative care, including vaccinations, well-woman exams, and mammograms and other cancer screenings (HHS, 2022b).

CONSUMER PROTECTION PROVISIONS

The ACA reformed the health insurance market with many consumer protection provisions. The reforms include eliminating lifetime coverage limits, restricting annual limits, prohibiting or rescinding coverage unless fraud is proven, and eliminating preexisting condition exclusions intended to provide immediate benefits to consumers with higher-than-average health care needs who were facing difficulties in receiving and paying for health care due to limits on coverage or loss of coverage. Other reforms in this category include giving patients the right to select the health care provider of their choice, appeal the denials or decisions made by their health insurance plans, and access emergency care even if out-of-network (ACA, 2010d).

OBTAINING AND RENEWING HEALTH INSURANCE

The ACA also reformed the ways for individuals to obtain health insurance coverage. The former practice of health insurers being allowed to discriminate and deny coverage based on perceived high risk or likeliness to use the insurance was eliminated. Before this reform, individuals with chronic health conditions requiring long-term management of diseases like cardiac diseases, HIV, diabetes, or cancer were often unable to purchase insurance if they did not have access to employer-sponsored insurance. This practice was especially detrimental to women of childbearing age, as they are more likely to incur significant medical expenses during pregnancy, childbirth, and postpartum. Even if women were allowed to purchase insurance, pregnancy was considered a preexisting condition; hence, coverage was denied. ACA prohibited insurers from such discriminatory practices and required them to provide coverage to anyone who applied, regardless of all factors, including gender and health status.

Additionally, ACA also required insurers to guarantee the renewability of health insurance, despite any health issues that may have been discovered and covered before the renewal. For example, before the ACA, if an insured person was diagnosed with cancer and received treatment in the past coverage period (usually a year-long period), they could be denied coverage renewal for a new coverage period based on their past insurance usage. This would cause individuals to be left uninsured and unable to access care without paying substantially higher out-of-pocket costs. This loophole was closed by the ACA (2010d).

Health Insurance Cost and Variations

The ACA (2010d) protected consumers from increased premiums paid to health insurers based on their health status, insurance usage, or perceived risks. Limitations and conditions under which insurance premiums can be adjusted were defined as follows:

- Individual vs. family enrollment. Insurers may adjust premium rates based on the number of family members enrolled in the plan. More qualifying family members added to the plan would mean higher premiums.
- Geographical areas and cost of living/care can affect the premium rates.
- Older adults can be charged higher rates, but it is limited to no more than three times what younger adults are charged under the same plan.
- Tobacco users may be charged up to 1.5 times more than insureds who refrain from tobacco use.

TRANSPARENCY

The ACA required all health insurance plans to provide standardized and easy-to-read information on the summary of benefits and coverage (SBC). The required information on the SBC is the plan's main features, covered benefits, any limitations or exclusions on coverage, cost-sharing and copay requirements, and whether the plan meets minimum essential coverage standards. This standardized information is intended to make comparing and picking a health insurance plan simpler and more transparent for buyers. Additionally, the SBC must include examples of coverage for hypothetical health issues. The current standard SBC sheet includes costs covered by the health insurance plan and the cost to the consumers for normal childbirth and type 2 diabetes. The SBC must also include uniform and easy-to-understand definitions of common insurance-related terms, like "deductibles," "out-of-pocket costs," "copays," and so on. These provisions were developed to help consumers make informed decisions without being confused by the jargon.

POST-INTRODUCTION ANALYSIS

In the 12 years, following the introduction of the ACA, Americans and health care systems saw many improvements. Some effects the ACA had on health care include but are not limited to the following:

- The policy expanded health insurance coverage to 32 million previously uninsured people in the United States. In 2016, 5 years after ACA was implemented, the uninsured rate in the United States was at 9%, an all-time low at the time. In 2021, uninsured rates were 6.6% and 12.7% in states with expanded Medicaid and those without expansion, respectively. Nationwide, the uninsured rate ranged from 2.5%, in Massachusetts, to 18.0%, in Texas (U.S. Census Bureau, 2022).
- The focus of health care shifted from treatment to prevention by requiring all private health insurance plans (except grandfathered plans) to provide coverage for preventative services without any cost to the insured. The required preventative services are (a) evidence-based services rated A or B by the U.S. Preventive Services Task Force (USPSTF), (b) routine immunizations recommended by the Advisory Committee on Immunization Practices for both adult and child

immunizations against influenza, meningitis, hepatitis A and B, human papillomavirus (HPV), measles, mumps, rubella, and varicella (chicken pox), or (c) preventive services for children and youth recommended by the Health Resources and Services Administration's Bright Futures Project, including immunizations; behavioral and development assessments; and screening for autism, vision and hearing impairment, tuberculosis, and certain genetic diseases (ACA, 2010e). By 2014, 76 million adults and children had received no-cost coverage for preventive health services since the ACA preventive services coverage rules had taken effect (Burke & Simmons, 2014).

- Women's preventative and sexual health services became accessible with no cost sharing. Services include well-woman visits, all FDA-approved contraceptives, breastfeeding support and supplies, mammograms, screenings for cervical cancer, prenatal care, screenings for domestic violence, Human Immunodeficiency Virus (HIV) screening, and sexually transmitted infections (STI) counseling (Health Resources and Services Administration [HRSA], 2022a). Approximately 58 million women currently benefit from this expanded provision and 37 million children have access to preventative services (Office of the Assistant Secretary of Planning and Evaluation, 2022). The only exception is that nonprofit religious organizations and some religious for-profit organizations are allowed to deny coverage for contraceptives, as decided by the Supreme Court in *Burwell v. Hobby Lobby* (2014).
- New provisions were made for states to expand Medicaid eligibility up to 138% of the FPL Level ($17,774 for an individual; $36,570 for a family of four) and categorical

requirements that had prevented many low-income people from being able to enroll in the program were removed. Not all states have expanded their Medicaid programs, notably including Texas. However, as of March 2022, 38 states and Washington DC, have expanded Medicaid to expand coverage for their residents, leading to decreased health disparities and improved health outcomes for women of color and families (CMS, 2020a; HHS, 2022b).

- The legislation provided $25 million in grants to benefit nearly 110,000 expectant and young parents in 32 states and seven tribal organizations via the Pregnancy Assistance Fund Program (PAFP; Office of Population Affairs, 2020). Additionally, it allocated $4.7 billion to support home visiting services to expectant parents and those with young children living in communities with greater barriers to achieving positive maternal health outcomes (Office of Early Childhood Development, 2022). HRSA provided over 7.2 million home visits between 2012 and 2020 (HRSA, 2022b).
- The Center for Medicare and Medicaid Innovation (CMS Innovation Center) was established with the aim of innovating payment and service models that improve patient outcomes while lowering costs for those insured by Medicare, Medicaid, and the Children's Health Insurance Program (CHIP; CMS, 2022a).
- The policy made essential medications more affordable for Medicare beneficiaries by closing the Medicare Part D prescription coverage gap, or "donut hole."

Funding, Cost Containment Measures, and Impact on Health Care Costs

As with any other legislation, funding is the most important aspect. The previously discussed monetary appropriations and allocations must come from federal or state government resources. The ACA came with a costly price tag: a 10-year cost estimate of $940 billion in 2010. In 2012, the Congressional Budget Office (CBO) estimated a cost of $1.8 trillion for the 10 years between 2012–2022, partially offset by $510 billion in receipts and cost savings (CBO, 2012). The CBO updated the price tag as more information and data became available. In 2015, it was estimated that the cost for 2015–2015 would be $1.207 trillion (CBO, 2015).

While the price tag seems hefty, it is crucial to understand that the ACA helped reduce health care spending growth and price inflation. In 2015, due in part to the ACA, health care spending grew at the slowest rate since 1960. Meanwhile, health care price inflation is at its lowest rate in 50 years (Assistant Secretary for Planning and Evaluation, 2022).

A diversified portfolio funds the ACA. Some sources include a Medicare investment tax, a 3.8% tax on investment incomes over $200,000/individual or $250,000/couple; a health insurance tax, an annual fee on health insurers; a tanning tax, a 10% tax on tanning services; a Cadillac tax, a 40% tax on high-cost health insurance; a Medicare payroll tax; a brand name drug tax, a 2.3% medical device tax; individual mandates with a penalty for not having health insurance and a similar employer mandate for not offering health insurance; and other sources (Internal Revenue Service [IRS], 2010; American College of Physicians, 2013; Green, 2021; IRS, 2022). Some of these provisions, including the Cadillac tax, were later repealed, but ACA continues to take cost containment measures to improve health care for Americans while keeping costs low.

Cost-Containment: Medicare

On the Medicare side, some cost-containment provisions that impacted the financial aspects of health care are restructuring Medicare Advantage payments as variable based on fee-for-service (FFS) rates, with higher payments for areas with low FFS rates and lower payments (95% of FFS) for areas with high FFS rates, providing bonuses to Medicare Advantage health plans receiving four or more stars on a 5-star rating system, double bonuses for qualifying plans in qualifying areas, penalties and partial paybacks for plans with medical loss ratio (MLR) of less than 85% (Patient Protection and ACA, 2010a). MLR is the share of total health care premiums spent on medical claims and efforts to improve the quality of care. Furthermore, the ACA reduced the annual market basket updates for inpatient hospitals, home health, skilled nursing facilities, hospice, and other Medicare providers and adjusted for productivity (ACA, 2010b). ACA also froze the threshold for Medicare Part B income-related premiums and reduced the Medicare Part D premium subsidy for those with incomes above $85,000/individual and $170,000/couple (ACA, 2010c). Other cost-containment measures include establishing an Independent Payment Advisory Board, comprising 15 members, which may submit legislative proposals with recommendations on reducing the per capita rate of growth of Medicare spending if it exceeds a target growth rate; reducing Medicare disproportionate share hospital (DSH) payments by 75% initially and subsequently increasing payments based on the percentage of the population uninsured and the amount of uncompensated care provided; eliminating the Medicare Improvement Fund; allowing accountable care organizations (ACOs) that meet quality standards to share in the cost savings they achieve for the Medicare program as a means to incentivize quality and evidence-based practice while reducing costs; and reducing Medicare payments to hospitals to account for preventable hospital readmissions and hospital-acquired conditions (Kaiser Family Foundation [KFF], 2013).

Cost-Containment: Medicaid

Similar to the Medicare cost-containment measures, reforms in the Medicaid program included prohibiting federal payments to states for Medicaid services required as a result of health-care-acquired conditions, increasing Medicaid drug rebate percentage for brand name drugs (with exceptions) to help to offset the federal and state costs of prescription drugs dispensed to Medicaid patients, and reducing aggregate Medicaid disproportionate share hospitals (DSH) allotments by imposing the largest reductions for states with the lowest percentages of uninsured and the smallest reductions for low-DSH states (KFF, 2013). DSHs are hospitals that provide health care to a disproportionate number of uninsured, indigent, and Medicaid patients. These facilities, called safety net hospitals, include public and private hospitals, children's hospitals, university hospital systems, and long-term mental health care institutions. The DSH program has become a critical funding source for the substantial costs of uncompensated care provided by safety net hospitals (Texas Legislative Council, 2003).

HEALTH CARE POLICY AND COVID-19

The COVID-19 pandemic brought forth the need for robust and timely health care policies. The accelerated timeline to create legislation and its enactment by regulatory agencies proved an important factor in addressing the public health crisis. In April 2020, the Centers for Medicare and Medicaid Services (CMS) issued regulatory waivers and rule changes during the pandemic to protect the public's health (CMS, 2020b, 2020c, 2020d). Some noteworthy efforts included the following:

- Eliminating the Medicare requirement for COVID-19 tests and certain other FDA-approved serology tests for a COVID-19 diagnosis to be ordered by a prescriber. Full coverage of COVID-19 tests was provided, with no cost to the insured.
- Allowing hospital outpatient departments to relocate off-site to increase hospitals' bed capacity

- Supporting the health care workforce by reducing administrative burden and allowing community mental health centers to offer partial hospitalization and other mental health services to clients in the safety of their homes
- Expanding telehealth services by including physical therapists, occupational therapists, and speech–language pathologists as telehealth providers, waiving the video requirements on behavioral health and patient education visits, and reimbursing audio-only visits to match the reimbursement for similar office/outpatient visits.
- Delaying Merit-based Incentive Payment System (MIPS) Qualified Clinical Data Registry (QCDR) measure approval criteria by 1 year.

The Families First Coronavirus Response Act (Public Law No. 116-127, 2020) is another important legislation passed into law. The act provided supplemental emergency funding, exempting federal agencies from discretionary spending limits to respond to the pandemic. The U.S. Department of Agriculture (USDA) was authorized to provide increased benefits under the Special Supplemental Nutrition Program for Women, Infants, and Children (WIC) and the Emergency Food Assistance Program (TEFAP), including emergency benefits for families with children who would be eligible for free or reduced-price lunch programs if their schools were not closed.

Emergency family and medical leave were expanded to permit employees to take public health emergency leave to care for their child during a COVID-19 school closures. Employers with fewer than 500 employees were required to provide up to 12 weeks of paid leave for an employee who could not work due to childcare burden. Full-time employees received 80 hours of paid sick leave, usable immediately, and part-time employees received paid sick leave, equaling their average hours worked in a 2-week period. Unemployment benefits were expanded. Tax credits against payroll taxes were provided to support paid sick and family leaves and included tax credits for self-employed individuals.

The act also appropriated the Public Health and Social Services Emergency Fund to support the National Disaster Medical System. The appropriation aimed to reimburse COVID-19 diagnostic testing and services to those without health insurance. Medicare, Medicaid, Medicare Advantage plans, Department of Defense (i.e., TRICARE), Department of Veterans Affairs, Indian Health Services, and private insurers were required to cover testing for COVID-19 and related visits to health care providers without imposing cost-sharing (e.g., deductibles, coinsurance, or copayments) for the duration of the public health emergency. Emergency use authorizations (EUA) were issued for diagnostic tools for detecting or diagnosing COVID-19, personal respiratory protective devices, and other medical devices for use during the COVID-19 outbreak (FDA, 2020).

Expanding the scope of practice of nurse practitioners was an unprecedented regulation that allowed advanced practice registered nurses (APRNs) to practice to the full extent of their training and education. The COVID-19 pandemic led to drastic increases in staffing shortages and expanded workloads for clinical health care professionals. Government officials called for retired nurse practitioners, physicians, nurses, and other medical professionals to return to the workforce and assist frontline staff. Collaborative practice agreement requirements were temporarily waived at the state level to allow independent practice authority to APRNs. Only seven restricted-practice states did not fully or partially waive the collaborative requirements. Nurse practitioners were authorized to order select diagnostic tests and medications that previously required a physician's orders. The Coronavirus Aid, Relief, and Economic Security Act (CARES Act; H.R. 748) permanently permitted nurse practitioners to order and provide Medicare-eligible home health services, which mitigated the spread of COVID-19 by keeping vulnerable patients at home.

Many barriers to independent practice were waived temporarily, expanding the scope of practice regulations. When the U.S. health care system struggled to provide care adequately and experienced a severe shortage of providers, APRNs proved indispensable. Research suggests nurse practitioners have long provided equitable care compared to their physician counterparts (Buerhaus et al., 2018; Kurtzman & Barnow, 2017; Woo et al., 2017).

CHAPTER SUMMARY

The study of policy encompasses both artistic finesse and scientific rigor. Nursing, an art in itself, employs scientific methodologies to shape policies. Policies serve as guiding instruments for specific domains, including public policy that impacts various processes. Health policy, a transformative force, encompasses laws and regulations that directly influence patient care. Nurses, with their understanding of policy implications, are pivotal in advocating for change, particularly at the grassroots level. Advocacy encompasses problem identification, solution proposal and associated costs, assessing the impact of the proposal on systems and care access, and defining the ultimate objectives. Thorough evaluation, even for partially implemented policies, remains indispensable. Notable examples, such as the Clinton Health Care Initiative and EMTALA, underscore the potency of bipartisan policy endeavors.

Health care policy plays a decisive role in shaping the health care landscape and influencing public health and well-being. Policies enacted at various tiers influence access, coverage, costs, and health care delivery. Noteworthy illustrations include the Affordable Care Act, which successfully curtailed the uninsured rate, and the No Surprises Act, designed to tackle unexpected medical billing. HIPAA's enactment ensured patient data privacy, while policies aimed at curbing tobacco sales significantly reduced smoking rates. Impactful ramifications are also evident in immunization and rural health care policies. The interplay between policy, governance, and localized responses, exemplified in scenarios such as Iowa, underscores the intricate facets of policy implementation and its far-reaching consequences.

Nurses are armed with local engagement, committee involvement, and research-backed advocacy, which gives them considerable influence over health care policy. Paramount among their concerns is health care access, with policies such as the ACA sculpting the landscape. The ACA's objectives encompassed coverage expansion, disparity reduction, and health care quality enhancement. Despite progress, lingering health indicators persist as challenges, especially among marginalized communities and low-income groups. The ACA's provisions encompassed eliminating preexisting condition denials, expanding Medicaid, and enabling young adults to remain on parental insurance. Its broader aims include enhancing health care accessibility and affordability as well as addressing systemic disparities.

The ACA ushered in consumer protection provisions that fundamentally transformed the health insurance realm, abolishing lifetime coverage limitations, forbidding preexisting condition exclusions, and conferring the right to select health care providers and challenge insurance decisions. The ACA's transformative reach extended to insurance acquisition and renewal, eradicating discrimination grounded in perceived risk and ensuring renewal guarantees. Efforts to mitigate premium increases tied to health status gained ground—as did the introduction of transparency via standardized benefit summaries. In the 12 years following its introduction, the ACA has led to expanded coverage, a shift toward prevention, bolstered women's health services, Medicaid enlargement, innovative health care models, and the closure of coverage gaps.

The ACA's fiscal underpinnings and cost containment strategies sought to enhance health care while reining in escalating costs. Funding for the ACA emerged from sources encompassing the Medicare investment tax, health insurance tax, and penalties for noncompliance. Evident strides were made in restraining health care expenditure growth and inflation. Cost containment endeavors extended to both Medicare and Medicaid, including payment restructuring, incentivizing providers, and moderating payment updates. The tumultuous landscape of the COVID-19 pandemic ushered in rapid health care policy modifications, notably expanded telehealth access, emergency family leave provisions, and amplified scope of practice for health care professionals, notably nurse practitioners. These adaptations effectively tackled the challenges posed by the crisis, fostering more efficient health care delivery.

Food for Thought

1. In what significant ways has the ACA impacted health care?
2. How has the ACA benefited different populations?

KEY POINTS

- Policies guide actions and influence public processes, including health policy.
- Health policy aims to create significant changes and encompasses patient care laws and rules.
- Advocacy involves defining problems, proposing solutions, assessing impacts, and clarifying goals.
- Evaluation is crucial for assessing the effectiveness of policies, even partially implemented ones.

- Health care policy shapes the health care system, impacting access, coverage, costs, and delivery.
- State preemption during the COVID-19 pandemic highlights the interplay between policy, governance, and local responses.
- Nurses influence health care policy through local engagement, committee participation, and research-backed advocacy.
- The COVID-19 pandemic prompted rapid health care policy changes, including telehealth expansion, emergency family leave, and scope of practice expansions for health care professionals, especially nurse practitioners.

ACTIVITIES

1. Reflect on a time when you encountered a challenge in patient care you believe could have been addressed by a policy change. What steps could nurses take to advocate for such changes?
2. Imagine you are a policymaker faced with the challenge of improving access to health care for underserved populations. What considerations would you take into account when proposing policy solutions?

Group Activity: The Policy Quest Game

1. Start your journey by selecting a character and setting (e.g., urban hospital, rural clinic, or research institute).
2. You will encounter different scenarios representing real-world policy challenges. Each scenario presents a description of the situation and multiple options for action.
3. Read the scenario carefully, and then choose an action you believe aligns with effective policy development, advocacy, or implementation. Your choices will impact the story's outcome.
4. After making a choice, you will receive feedback on the consequences of your decision. Did your choice lead to positive change, setbacks, or unforeseen challenges?

5. As you progress, you'll accumulate points based on the quality of your decisions and their impact on health care policy and patient care.

Scenarios

1. **policy advocacy:** You encounter a lack of access to mental health services in your community. Do you choose to collaborate with local organizations to advocate for increased funding for mental health programs or focus on providing direct care to your patients?
2. **policy implementation:** You are tasked with implementing a new patient data privacy policy in your health care facility. Do you prioritize staff training, seek patient input, or emphasize strict enforcement?
3. **health care disparities:** You learn that underserved communities in your area face significant health disparities. Will you engage in research to gather data supporting policy changes or lead community health education initiatives?
4. **emergency response:** A pandemic strikes, leading to an overwhelming number of patients. Do you advocate for the flexible scope of practice regulations to increase health care workforce or focus on managing immediate patient needs?
5. **patient-centered care:** A policy proposes cutting funds for preventive care services. Will you work with a multidisciplinary team to present evidence on the long-term cost savings of prevention or concentrate on your current patient workload?

Outcome

At the end of the game, your accumulated points reflect your ability to navigate health care policy challenges effectively. Reflect on your decisions and their outcomes and consider how your choices align with your personal values and beliefs as a nurse.

REFERENCES

Agency for Health care Research and Quality. (2013). 2012 *National health care disparities report.* http://archive.ahrq.gov/research/findings/nhqrdr/nhdr12/index.html

Altman, D. (2016). The Affordable Care Act's little-noticed success: cutting the uninsured rate. *The Wall Street Journal/Kaiser Family Foundation.* https://www.kff.org/uninsured/perspective/the-affordable-care-acts-little-noticed-success-cutting-the-uninsured-rate/

American Bar Association. (2021). What is an executive order? https://www.americanbar.org/groups/public_education/publications/teaching-legal-docs/what-is-an-executive-order-/

American College of Physicians. (2013). *How is the patient protection and Affordable Care Act (ACA) funded?* https://www.acponline.org/system/files/documents/advocacy/where_we_stand/assets/i2-how-is-the-aca-funded.pdf

Antos, J. R., & Capretta, J. C. (2020). *The ACA: Trillions? Yes. A revolution? No.* https/doi.org/10.1377/forefront.20200406.93812

Assistant Secretary for Planning and Evaluation. (2022). *The Affordable Care Act and its accomplishments: Briefing book.* https://aspe.hhs.gov/sites/default/files/documents/18cd655222dc3de64866b269143731ce/aca-briefing-book-aspe-03-2022.pdf

Buerhaus, P., Perloff, J., Clarke, S., O'Reilly-Jacob, M., Zolotusky, G., & DesRoches, C. M. (2018). Quality of primary care provided to Medicare beneficiaries by nurse practitioners and physicians. *Medical Care, 56*(6), 484–490. https://doi.org/10.1097/MLR.0000000000000908

Burwell v. Hobby Lobby Stores, Inc. :: 573 U.S. 682 (2014).

Burke, A., & Simmons, A. (2014). *Increased coverage of preventive services with zero cost sharing under the Affordable Care Act.* Office of the Assistant Secretary for Planning and Evaluation, Department of Health and Human Services. http://aspe.hhs.gov/health/reports/2014/preventiveservices/ib_preventiveservices.pdf

Centers for Medicare & Medicaid Services. (2023). *National health expenditure data.* https://www.cms.gov/research-statistics-data-and-systems/statistics-trends-and-reports/nationalhealthexpenddata/nhe-fact-sheet

Centers for Medicare and Medicaid Services. (2020a). *Medicaid expansion and what it means for you.* https://www.health care.gov/medicaid-chip/medicaid-expansion-and-you/

Centers for Medicare and Medicaid Services. (2020b). *COVID-19 emergency declaration blanket waivers for health care providers.* https://www.cms.gov/files/document/summary-covid-19-emergency-declaration-waivers.pdf

Centers for Medicare and Medicaid Services. (2020c). *Trump administration issues second round of sweeping changes to support U.S. health care system during COVID-19 pandemic.* https://www.cms.gov/newsroom/press-releases/trumpadministration-issues-second-round-sweeping-changes-support-us-health care-systemduring-covid

Centers for Medicare and Medicaid Services. (2020d). *Medicare and Medicaid Programs, basic health program, and exchanges; additional policy and regulatory revisions in response to the COVID-19 public health emergency and delay of certain reporting requirements for the skilled nursing facility quality reporting program.* https://www.cms.gov/files/document/covidmedicare-and-medicaid-ifc2.pdf

Centers for Medicare and Medicaid Services. (2022a). *The CMS innovation center.* https://innovation.cms.gov/

Centers for Medicare and Medicaid Services. (2022b). *No surprises: Understand your rights against surprise medical bills.* https://www.cms.gov/newsroom/fact-sheets/no-surprises-understand-your-rights-against-surprise-medical-bills

Central Intelligence Agency. (2022a). *The world factbook. 2013 estimates of infant mortality rates worldwide.* https://www.cia.gov/the-world-factbook/field/infant-mortality-rate/country-comparison

Central Intelligence Agency. (2022b). *The world factbook. Life expectancy at birth.* https://www.cia.gov/the-world-factbook/field/life-expectancy-at-birth/country-comparison

Congressional Budget Office. (2012). *Updated estimates for the insurance coverage provisions of the Affordable Care Act.* https://www.cbo.gov/sites/default/files/49973-Updated_Budget_Projections.pdf

Congressional Budget Office. (2015). *Updated budget projections 2015–2025.* https://www.cbo.gov/sites/default/files/49973-Updated_Budget_Projections.pdf

Constitution of the United States. (1787). *Article VI supreme law.* https://constitution.congress.gov/constitution/article-6/

Ducey, D. A. (2020). State of Arizona executive order 2020–12 prohibiting the closure of essential services. *Arizona Governor.* https://azgovernor.gov/sites/default/files/eo_2021_0.pdf

Healthy People 2030. (n.d.). https://health.gov/healthypeople

Hoadley, J., Alker, J. & Holmes, M. (2018). *Health insurance coverage in small towns and rural America: The role of Medicaid expansion.* Rural Health Policy Project, Georgetown University Health Policy Institute: Center for Children and Families. https://ccf.georgetown.edu/topic/rural-health/

Institute of Medicine. (2008). Evidence-based medicine and the changing nature of health care: 2007 IOM annual meeting summary. *National Academies Press; 7,* Policy changes to improve the value we need from health care. https://www.ncbi.nlm.nih.gov/books/NBK52830/

Internal Revenue Service. (2010). *Affordable Care Act tax provisions.* https://www.irs.gov/affordable-care-act/affordable-care-act-tax-provisions

Internal Revenue Service. (2022). *Affordable Care Act Provision 9010: Health insurance providers fee.* https://www.irs.gov/businesses/corporations/affordable-care-act-provision-9010

Kaiser Family Foundation. (2013). *Summary of the Affordable Care Act.* https://www.kff.org/health-reform/fact-sheet/summary-of-the-affordable-care-act/

Kirkham, C. (2020). *Trump administration restricts some e-cigarette flavors.* Reuters. https://www.reuters.com/article/us-usa-vaping/trump-administration-restricts-some-e-cigarette-flavors-idUSKBN1Z11B7

Kurtzman, E. T., & Barnow, B. S. (2017). A comparison of nurse practitioners, physician assistants, and primary care physicians' patterns of practice and quality of care in health centers. *Medical Care, 55*(6), 615–622. https://doi.org/10.1097/MLR.0000000000000689

Levy, D. T., Tam, J., Kuo, C., Fong, G. T., & Chaloupka, F. (2018). The impact of implementing tobacco control policies: The 2017 tobacco control policy scorecard. *Journal of Public Health Management and Practice, 24*(5), 448–457. https/doi.org/10.1097/PHH.0000000000000780

McKeon, J. (2022). *How new federal, state laws impact health care data privacy.* Health IT Security. https://healthitsecurity.com/features/how-new-federal-state-laws-impact-health care-data-privacy

Mervosh, S., Bogel-Burroughs, N., McDonnell Nieto del Rio, G., & Arango, T. (2020). How Iowa's governor went from dismissing mask mandates to ordering one herself. *The New York Times.* https://www.nytimes.com/2020/11/18/us/coronavirus-mask-mandate-iowa-reynolds.html

Mervosh, S. & Healy, J. (2020). Holdout states resist calls for stay-at-home orders: 'What are you waiting for?' *The New York Times.* https://www.nytimes.com/2020/04/03/us/coronavirus-states-without-stay-home.html

Motacki, K., & Burke, K. M. (2017). *Nursing delegation and management of patient care* (2nd ed.). Elsevier, Inc.

National Conference of State Legislators. (2020). *Improving rural health: State policy options for increasing access to care.* https://www.ncsl.org/health/improving-rural-health

Office of the Assistant Secretary of Planning and Evaluation. (2022). *Access to preventive services without cost-sharing: Evidence from the Affordable Care Act.* https://aspe.hhs.gov/reports/aca-preventive-services-without-cost-sharing

Office of Early Childhood Development. (2022). *Tribal maternal, infant, and early childhood home visiting.* https://www.acf.hhs.gov/ecd/tribal/tribal-home-visiting

Office of Population Affairs. (2020). *Pregnancy assistance fund program.* https://opa.hhs.gov/grant-programs/pregnancy-assistance-fund

Patient Protection and Affordable Care Act. (2010a). State flexibility to establish alternative programs Sec. 1331 Ø42 U.S.C. 18051. State flexibility to establish basic health programs for low-income individuals not eligible for Medicaid, Part 4, Section II (B) (b). *Patient Protection and Affordable Care Act Health-Related Portions of the Health Care and Education Reconciliation Act of 2010.* http://housedocs.houco.gov/onorgyoommoroo/ppaoaoon.pdf

Patient Protection and Affordable Care Act. (2010b). Quality reporting for long-term care hospitals, inpatient rehabilitation hospitals, and hospice programs. Sec 1814 U.S.C. 1395f(i)). *Patient Protection and Affordable Care Act Health-Related Portions of the Health Care and Education Reconciliation Act of 2010.* http://housedocs.house.gov/energycommerce/ppacacon.pdf

Patient Protection and Affordable Care Act. (2010c). Reducing Part D premium subsidy for high-income beneficiaries; Income-related increase in Part D premium, Sec. 3308. (A) *Patient Protection and Affordable Care Act Health-Related Portions of the Health Care and Education Reconciliation Act of 2010.* http://housedocs.house.gov/energycommerce/ppacacon.pdf

Patient Protection and Affordable Care Act (2010d). Part 147—Health insurance reform requirements for the group and individual health insurance markets; 42 U.S.C. 300gg through 300gg-63, 300gg-91, 300gg-92, and 300gg-111 through 300gg-139, as amended, and section 3203, Pub. L. 116-136, 134 Stat. 281. *Patient Protection and Affordable Care Act Health-Related Portions of the Health Care and Education Reconciliation Act of 2010.* http://housedocs.house.gov/energycommerce/ppacacon.pdf

Patient Protection and Affordable Care Act (2010e). Title 45—Public Welfare Subtitle A—Department of health and human services, Subchapter b—Requirements relating to health care access, Part 147—Health insurance reform requirements for the group and individual health insurance markets, Section 147.130—Coverage of preventive health services. *Patient Protection and Affordable Care Act Health-Related Portions of the Health Care and Education Reconciliation Act of 2010.* http://housedocs.house.gov/energycommerce/ppacacon.pdf

Pollitz, K., Lopes, L., Kearney, A., Rae, M., Cox, C., Fehr, R. & Rousseau, D. (2022). US statistics on surprise medical billing. *The Journal of the American Medical Association, 323*(6), 498. https/doi.org/10.1001/jama.2020.0065

Rogers, S. (2022). What is health care policy and why is it important? *Promed Certifications.* https://promedcert.com/blog/what-is-health care-policy-and-why-is-it-important/

Rutkow, L., Vernick, J., Hodge, J., & Teret, S. (2008). Preemption and the obesity epidemic: State and local menu labeling laws and the nutrition labeling and education act. *Journal of Law, Medicine & Ethics, 36*(4), 772–789. https/doi.org/10.1111/j.1748-720X.2008.00337.x

Schneider, E. C., Shah, A., Doty, M. M., Tikkanen, R., Fields, K., & Williams, R. D. (2021). Mirror, mirror 2021—Reflecting poorly: Health care in the U.S.

compared to other high-income countries. *Commonwealth Fund.* https://doi.org/10.26099/01DV-H208

Texas Legislative Council. (2003). *Disproportionate Share Hospital (DSH) program: Your questions answered.* https://tlc.texas.gov/docs/policy/dshprogram.pdf

The HIPAA Guide. (2017). *Why was HIPAA created?* https://www.hipaaguide.net/why-was-hipaa-created/

The HIPAA Journal. (2023). *HIPAA history.* https://www.hipaajournal.com/hipaa-history/

The White House, Office of the Press Secretary. (2009). *Remarks by the President to the annual conference of the American Medical Association.* https://obamawhitehouse.archives.gov/the-press-office/remarks-president-annual-conference-american-medical-association

Tolbert, J., Drake, P. & Damico, A. (2022). Key facts about the uninsured population. *Kaiser Family Foundation.* https://www.kff.org/uninsured/issue-brief/key-facts-about-the-uninsured-population/

U.S. Census Bureau. (2022). *Decline in share of people without health insurance driven by increase in public coverage in 36 states.* https://www.census.gov/library/stories/2022/09/uninsured-rate-declined-in-28-states.html#:~:text=State%20Differences%20in%20the%20Uninsured%20Rate%20in%202021&text=In%202021%2C%20the%20uninsured%20rate%20was%206.6%25%20in%20expansion%20states,had%20not%20expanded%20Medicaid%20eligibility

U.S. Department of Health and Human Services. (2022a). *About the Affordable Care Act.* https://www.hhs.gov/health care/about-the-aca/index.html#:~:text=Make%20affordable%20health%20insurance%20available,below%20138%25%20of%20the%20FPL

U.S. Department of Health and Human Services. (2022b). *Fact sheet: Celebrating the Affordable Care Act: 12 years of advancing health equity for all Americans.* https://www.hhs.gov/health care/about-the-aca/index.html#:~:text=Make%20affordable%20health%20insurance%20available,below%20138%25%20of%20the%20FPL

U.S. Food and Drug Administration. (2019). *Trump administration combating epidemic of youth e-cigarette use with plan to clear market of unauthorized, non-tobacco-flavored e-cigarette products*. https://www.fda.gov/news-events/press-announcements/trump-administration-combating-epidemic-youth-e-cigarette-use-plan-clear-market-unauthorized-non

U.S. Food and Drug Administration. (2020). *Coronavirus disease 2019 (COVID-19) emergency use authorizations for medical devices*. https://www.fda.gov/medical-devices/emergency-use-authorizations-medical-devices/coronavirus-disease-2019-covid-19-emergency-use-authorizations-medical-devices

U.S. Food and Drug Administration. (2022). *Results from the annual national youth tobacco survey*. https://www.fda.gov/tobacco-products/youth-and-tobacco/results-annual-national-youth-tobacco-survey?utm_campaign=ctp-

Woo, B. F. Y., Lee, J. X. Y., & Tam, W. W. S. (2017). The impact of the advanced practice nursing role on quality of care, clinical outcomes, patient satisfaction, and cost in the emergency and critical care settings: A systematic review. *Human Resources for Health, 15*(1), 63. https://doi.org/10.1186/s12960-017-0237-9

CHAPTER 9

Legal Parameters of Care and Practice

Kathleen Siders, Robert Coghlan III, and Aastha Krebs

OBJECTIVES

Upon completion of the chapter, the student will be able to

1. appraise the function of the consensus model
2. plan the necessary steps to obtain licensure within a state
3. compare the impact to practice of each level of APRN supervision

QUESTIONS/CHALLENGES

1. What is your scope of practice?
2. What are the continuing education requirements for APRNs in your state or country?
3. What type of supervision is required in your state or country?

INTRODUCTION

Completing an education program for preparation as a nurse practitioner (NP) is the first step toward the new role. Further actions are needed before the graduate is recognized as an advanced practice registered nurse (APRN) and granted the privilege of practice. This chapter elucidates the purpose and function of certification, licensure, and credentialling for the new NP.

Understanding the legal boundaries of practice alleviates missteps and stress when preparing for and beginning a new role as an NP. Several layers of laws, rules, policies, and regulations define the boundaries of the APRN. Health care systems and individual practices base their policies and procedures on local, state, and federal guidance. For safe practice, APRNs must understand where to find the guidance and how to apply it to the day-to-day practice of advanced nursing practice. The new role does not supplant the guidance of a registered nurse (RN). NPs must also adhere to all rules and regulations of an RN.

In addition, this chapter will discuss required NP supervision and health care ethics. With increased responsibility comes increased entanglement of competing interests. Health care resources are limited and competing interests lead to complex decision making through an ethical structure.

PRACTICE ACT

All 50 states and territories regulate the practice of nursing through individual nurse practice acts (NPAs). Before 1903, "nurse" was not a protected name; anyone could call themselves a nurse. In 1903, North Carolina passed a nurse registration law to protect and improve nursing practice. To increase the oversight of nurses, states created nursing regulatory bodies (NRB), often called boards of nursing (BON), to establish standards of safe nursing practice, issue licensing, and monitor nursing practice (Nursing Council of State Boards of Nursing [NCSBN], n.d.). By the 1970s, licensure was required in all states for all nurses, both registered and vocational/practical nurses (Russel, 2017).

NPAs protect the public and the nurse's right to practice (Russell, 2017). The BONs establish APRN Scope of Practice (SOP), rules, and regulations. Nursing boards are not responsible for protecting nurses but must protect the nursing professional's right and ability to practice. Each state has a unique NPA with commonalities, including "definitions, authority, power, and composition of a BON, educational program standards, and scope of nursing practice, types of titles and licenses, protection of titles, requirements for licensure, and grounds for disciplinary action, other violations, and possible remedies" (Russel, 2017). All NPAs describe the qualifications for licensure, titles nurses may go by, SOP, and actions taken for breaching the law (NCSBN, n.d.). Beyond the NPA, BONs establish rules and regulations carrying the full force and effect of law to guide nurses.

APRNs are responsible for knowing their state's NPA and published rules and regulations. All BONs publish this information on their websites. As with all professions, NPs must understand their legal obligations and boundaries. When NPs need clarity for a specific situation, they should contact and query their BON. Professional organizations like the American Association of Nurse Practitioners (AANP) and their respective state branches keep constituents aware of changing regulations. These organizations also closely follow legislation and rule/regulation changes, advocating for the profession and informing members. Most organizations' websites provide convenient platforms for members to communicate with government officials to advocate for NPs.

Advanced Practice Registered Nurses (APRNs) have more specialized education and training than RNs, which qualifies them to perform more complex and specialized tasks. APRN education typically involves a master's or doctoral degree, while RNs usually have an associate's or bachelor's degree. APRNs also need to have a valid RN license to practice.

APRNs have skills and abilities RNs must gain, due to their advanced education and training. APRNs can prescribe medication, diagnose and treat illnesses, and provide advanced patient care. They also have in-depth knowledge of a specific area of health care, such as mental health, geriatrics, or pediatrics. Additionally, many APRNs are trained to perform advanced medical procedures, such as invasive surgeries. Overall, APRNs can provide more advanced and specialized health care services than RNs due to their education and training in a specific area of health care.

The licensure requirements for APRNs (Advanced Practice Registered Nurses) vary by state but typically include the following:

- **graduate degree:** APRNs must hold a graduate degree in nursing, such as a master of science in nursing (MSN) or doctor of nursing practice (DNP).
- **RN licensure:** APRNs must hold a valid RN license in the state in which they plan to practice.
- **national certification:** APRNs must obtain national certification in their specialty area, such as family practice, pediatrics, or psychiatry.
- **clinical hours:** APRNs are required to complete a certain number of clinical hours before being eligible for national certification and state licensure.
- **state licensure:** APRNs must obtain a state license to practice in the state where they plan to work.
- **continuing education:** APRNs must complete continuing education to maintain their license and certification in their specialty area. (Figure 9.1)

Continuing education requirements for APRNs vary by state and specialty. In general, APRNs must complete a specific number of continuing education (CE) hours every 2 years to maintain

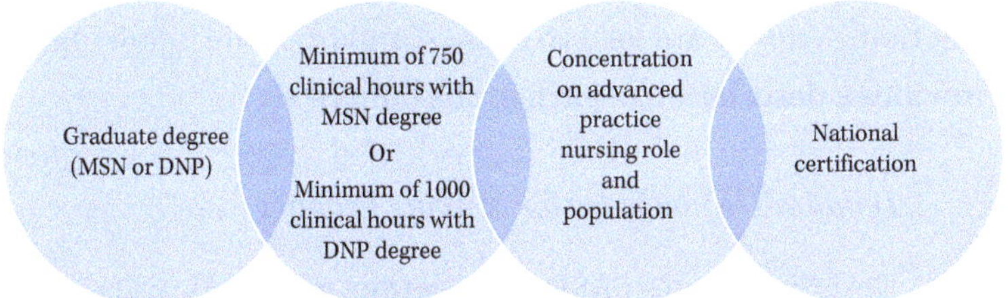

FIGURE 9.1 Primary requirements for APRN initial licensure.

their license and certification. For example, the National Council of State Boards of Nursing (NCSBN) recommends a minimum of 25 CE hours per year for APRNs. Some states require different amounts of CE hours, while others have no specific requirements. The types of CE hours needed may also vary depending on the APRN's specialty. For example, a family nurse practitioner may need CE in primary care, while a psychiatric-mental health nurse practitioner may need CE in mental health. APRNs may also be required to complete CE in specific topics, such as pharmacology or pain management. CE hours can include courses, workshops, conferences, or other educational activities that are relevant to their field of practice. APRNs may also be required to have a certain number of clinical hours or demonstrate proficiency in specific skills to maintain their license. Additionally, APRNs must adhere to ethical and professional standards set forth by their nursing board and may be subject to audits or continuing competency evaluations to ensure their continued competence and fitness to practice. APRNs should check with their state nursing board and certification organization for specific CE requirements.

The American Association of Colleges of Nursing (AACN) published a comprehensive list of nursing competencies, categorized in 10 domains, in 2021. The domains are common to all levels of nursing, and the competencies within the domains are divided into entry-level professional nursing education and advanced-level nursing education. Nursing education is currently tasked with implementing student evaluations based on these competencies.

Practicing APRNs are held to these standards. The following list provides a description of each of the domains:

> *Domain 1: Knowledge for Nursing Practice*
>
> Descriptor: Integration, translation, and application of established and evolving disciplinary nursing knowledge and ways of knowing, as well as knowledge from other disciplines, including a foundation in liberal arts and natural and social sciences. This distinguishes the practice of professional nursing and forms the basis for clinical judgment and innovation in nursing practice.
>
> *Domain 2: Person-Centered Care*
>
> Descriptor: Person-centered care focuses on the individual within multiple complicated contexts, including family and/or important others. Person-centered care is holistic, individualized, just, respectful, compassionate, coordinated, evidence-based, and developmentally appropriate. Person-centered care builds on a scientific body of knowledge that guides nursing practice regardless of specialty or functional area.
>
> *Domain 3: Population Health*
>
> Descriptor: Population health spans the health care delivery continuum from public health prevention to disease management of populations and describes collaborative activities with both traditional and non-traditional partnerships from affected communities, public health, industry, academia, health care, local government entities, and

others for the improvement of equitable population health outcomes.

Domain 4: Scholarship for Nursing Practice

Descriptor: The generation, synthesis, translation, application, and dissemination of nursing knowledge to improve health and transform health care.

Domain 5: Quality and Safety

Descriptor: Employment of established and emerging principles of safety and improvement science. Quality and safety, as core values of nursing practice, enhance quality and minimize the risk of harm to patients and providers through both system effectiveness and individual performance.

Domain 6: Interprofessional Partnerships

Descriptor: Intentional collaboration across professions and with care team members, patients, families, communities, and other stakeholders to optimize care, enhance the health care experience, and strengthen outcomes.

Domain 7: Systems-Based Practice

Descriptor: Responding to and leading within complex systems of health care. Nurses effectively and proactively coordinate resources to provide safe, quality, equitable care to diverse populations.

Domain 8: Informatics and Health Care Technologies

Descriptor: Information and communication technologies and informatics processes are used to provide care, gather data, form information to drive decision-making, and support professionals as they expand knowledge and wisdom for practice. Informatics processes and technologies are used to manage and improve the delivery of safe, high-quality, and efficient health care services in accordance with best practices and professional and regulatory standards.

Domain 9: Professionalism

Descriptor: Formation and cultivation of a sustainable professional nursing identity, accountability, perspective, collaborative disposition, and comportment that reflects nursing's characteristics and values.

Domain 10: Personal, Professional, and Leadership Development

Descriptor: Participation in activities and self-reflection that foster personal health, resilience, well-being, lifelong learning, and support the acquisition of nursing expertise and assertion of leadership. (AACN, 2021)

CONSENSUS MODEL

The contribution of APRNs to health care continues to expand in quantity and value. To decrease barriers to care, the NCSBN APRN Committee and the Advanced Practice Nursing Consensus Work Group collaborated to create and publish the Consensus Model of APRN Regulations in 2008. The purpose of this landmark document was to establish consensus on APRN practice throughout the states and territories of the United States. The document "defines APRN practice, describes the APRN regulatory model, identifies the titles to be used, defines specialty, describes the emergence of new roles and population foci, and presents strategies for implementation" (APRN Joint Dialogue Group, 2008, p. 5). Before the consensus model, states had varying population foci and definitions, creating difficulties for nurses applying for practice in another state.

The NCSBN and multiple nursing advocacy organizations are working toward further decreasing barriers to NP practice across state lines through the establishment of an APRN Compact. If enacted into law, the compact would allow an NP to practice with a multistate license in participating states. The APRN Compact would improve response during disasters or times of increased need for APRNs. The COVID-19 crisis exemplified the need for mobility across state lines. The APRN workforce numbers needed to fluctuate according to geographic areas and over time. A compact eliminates the need for paying for and maintaining multiple licenses. This is especially helpful for the frequent mobility of military spouses throughout the United States.

LEVELS OF SUPERVISION IN THE UNITED STATES

Each U.S. state and territory establishes levels of supervision for APRNs. Supervision is described as one health care professional overseeing another's practice. This relationship is represented by the terms "supervise, delegate, collaborate, and consult" in different legal documents (Ritter, 2018). The American Association of Nurse Practitioners (AANP, 2022) breaks supervision into three levels: full, reduced, and restricted. The AANP defines full practice authority (FPA) as allowing NPs to "evaluate, diagnose, order and interpret diagnostic tests; and initiate and manage treatments, including prescribing medication and controlled substances, under the exclusive licensure authority of the state board of nursing" (2022).

The AANP further points out that the National Academy of Medicine and the NCSBN each recommend FPA for NPs. In contrast, reduced practice is defined as reducing at least one aspect of NP practice and requiring a career-long regulated collaborative agreement with another health provider or limiting the setting of one or more elements of NP practice. Restricted practice mandates an NP must have career-long supervision, delegation, or team management by another health provider before providing patient care. Progress towards all states granting FPA to NPs has been slow. As of the writing of this chapter, 27 states have passed FPA legislation for NPs, with Utah most recently being added to this list.

Many states with FPA require a transition period of varying lengths of time for entry-to-practice NPs to work in collaboration with or under the supervision of an NP or MD (Taylor & Gilchrist, 2020). Some states stipulate that the supervising provider must be physically present in the same setting or within a geographic distance limit (Ritter, 2018). NPs are responsible for clearly knowing and understanding the various practice nuances mandated by their state's BON.

All health care providers work in collaboration within a team. Providers work within "networks," sometimes defined through their organizations and other times defined through the relationships individually created to provide comprehensive care successfully. This would include referral to or consultation with other providers. FPA provides autonomy but not isolation (Peacock, 2020). Autonomy respects the NP's knowledge and skills, including responsibly recognizing when to involve other health care team members to optimize care. Autonomy requires NPs to be self-aware to match their educational preparation, self-assess competencies, and any institutional or governmental SOP to determine their practice parameters.

Autonomy predicts job satisfaction for NPs (Peacock, 2020) but not necessarily empowerment, according to Peterson (2013), who studied the association of autonomy and empowerment with NPs in New Mexico. New Mexico has a more than 30 years of history with FPA. In Peterson's study, 40% of New Mexico's NPs reported practicing with physician oversight. Poghosyan et al. (2018) compared the reported work environment for NPs before and after gaining FPA in New York. This study concluded a significant work environment improvement for experienced and less experienced NPs. Poghosyan et al. (2022) conducted a cross-sectional survey of the work environment of NPs practicing in health care organizations in six states, equally divided amongst FPA, reduced authority, and restricted authority. The study found positive relationships between FPA and administration relations, independent practice and support, and professional visibility.

FPA for NPs increases access to care, especially in rural and underserved areas (Poghosyan et al., 2022; Plemmons et al., 2023; NAS). FPAs are also costly to maintain and sometimes hard to establish. One psychiatric mental health NP in Texas reports that in the face of a critically underserved population for adolescent psychiatric services in her area, she cannot secure a collaborating psychiatrist (personal communication, June, 2023). The U.S. supply of primary care physicians is rapidly falling behind the demand for their services (National Academy of Sciences, 2021). NPs are well positioned to aid in closing that gap and are more willing than physicians to practice in health provider shortage areas (Plemmons et al., 2023). Another suggested benefit of FPA is a decrease in health care costs without a decrease in quality outcomes (National Academy of Sciences, 2021). Along with restricted practice, outdated and unnecessary rules and regulations, such as the Center for Medicare Services' ban on NPs ordering diabetic shoes, restrict care and drive costs upwards due to unnecessary referrals for services clearly within the NP's scope of practice.

Several barriers to obtaining FPA exist in the remaining states. Despite many underserved communities throughout the states, NPs are often perceived as encroaching on their physician counterparts' territory and market share. Political influence from medicine outweighs that from the nursing community. Despite the imbalance of power, the tide is turning in favor of recognizing NPs potential to contribute to improving access to health care.

HEALTH CARE, LAW, AND ETHICS

Nurses have a unique perspective on health care and ethics. Haddad and Geiger (2022) state that "ethics" derives from the Greek word "ethos," meaning character. "Ethics" is defined as knowing the difference between right and wrong and is defined by our personal beliefs and values (Motacki, 2017). Ethics define a clear set of rules commonly accepted and followed, both personally and professionally. They define a society and how the society interacts with the surrounding world as well as direct the creation of policies and procedures that have a wider meaning beyond their respective authors. Gallup polls have rated nurses as the most ethical medical profession since they began including nurses in polls in 1998. Interestingly, ratings have changed for pharmacists and medical doctors since 2003 (Brenan, 2023). However, nurses remain rated higher, even when there is a decrease year over year. Nurses advocate for their patients without violating their patient's rights and beliefs or their personal beliefs and ethics. One of the hallmarks of any profession is the development of a core set of beliefs. These beliefs establish a standard for members of the profession to adhere to and hold others accountable. The American Nurses Association (2015) has developed the following nine provisions to guide nurses:

- **provision 1:** The nurse practices with compassion and respect for the inherent dignity of worth and unique attributes of every person.

- **provision 2:** The nurse's primary commitment is to the patient, whether an individual, family, group, community, or population.
- **provision 3:** The nurse promotes, advocates for, and protects the rights, health, and safety of the patient.
- **provision 4:** The nurse has authority, accountability, and responsibility for nursing practice; makes decisions; and takes action consistent with the obligation to provide optimal patient care.
- **provision 5:** The nurse owes the same duties to self as to others, including the responsibility to promote health and safety, preserve wholeness of character and integrity, maintain competence, and continue personal and professional growth.
- **provision 6:** The nurse, through individual and collective effort, establishes, maintains, and improves the ethical environment of the work setting and conditions of employment that are conducive to safe, quality health care.
- **provision 7:** The nurse, in all roles and settings, advances the profession through research and scholarly, inquiry, professional standards development, and the generations of both nursing and health policy.
- **provision 8:** The nurse collaborates with other health professionals and the public to protect human rights, promote health diplomacy, and reduce health disparities.
- **provision 9:** The profession of nursing, collectively through its professional organization, must articulate nursing values, maintain the profession's integrity, and integrate principles of social justice into nursing and health policy.

These nine provisions guide nursing members on conducting their activities related to direct patient care, advocacy for their patients, and changes to the medical system in operation. Participating in a practice that leads to an untoward outcome contrary to a patient's beliefs or clearly stated expected outcome is an ethical violation. Regardless of the program, nursing schools emphasize the importance of ethics in the curriculum, providing a guiding philosophy throughout students' careers.

History provides many examples of laws, rules, and regulations that would now be in violation of the ANA Code of Ethics for Nurses. Nurses who participated in the involuntary euthanasia of handicapped children and mentally ill adults in early 1940s Germany serve as an egregious example of ethical violation (Benedict, 1999). Later, during World War II, nurses actively engaged in experimentation, torture, killings, and brutal behavior towards those in custody by the Nazi Regime (Benedict, 1999). Nurses act ethically despite stress. Patients must be able to consent and approve of any treatment plan they are going to participate in. Nurses must ensure all patients are treated consistently, regardless of any racial, ethnic, religious, or financial concerns. Additionally, nurses must ensure that harm is not done to the patient by either withholding care of the patient, even after the patient has been given all the appropriate education. But it is also true that a nurse would be in violation of ethics if they provided care that was not authorized, directly or indirectly, either by the patient or their advocate. An example would be to either discontinue a care regimen or implement a care regimen the patient or their advocate did not request or authorize. There are occasions when a patient either does not wish to receive extensive life-extending care, or vice versa, in which case they do expect and have requested for everything possible be done to extend their life, regardless of the diagnosis or enhancement to care. The nurse must carry out the plan of care as written/ordered by the provider. However, the nurse could also discuss their concerns with the plan of care with the provider. There is always the process of bringing the concerns to their leadership and, if necessary (based on the policy of the institution), requesting an ethics consult. If the nurse feels their personal and professional ethics are violated, they must decide to either continue the care or turn it over to another nurse or health care provider. The nurse cannot simply abandon the patient, as that would cause the patient harm. This is known as the principle of "nonmaleficence," or avoiding actions that would cause harm to a patient (Haddad & Geiger, 2022).

CHAPTER SUMMARY

The APRN's roles and responsibilities continue to change. State boards of nursing; professional organizations, such as the AACN; and legislative bodies on local, state, and national levels establish scopes of practice. Each APRN is responsible for knowing their professional boundaries and staying abreast of shifting changes. Appreciating the history and evolvement of APRNs, including efforts to standardize the profession, such as the consensus model, informs advocacy efforts on behalf of the profession. As with any profession, APRNs work within ethical boundaries while providing care to the public.

Food for Thought

1. What are your thoughts on advanced directives?
2. How would you proceed in overcoming the barriers to full practice authority?

KEY POINTS

- Nursing regulatory bodies (NRBs), often called boards of nursing (BONs), establish standards of safe nursing practice, issue licensing, and monitor nursing practice certification.

- The APRN is responsible for knowing the BON's APRN scope of practice (SOP), rules, and regulations.
- The American Association of Colleges of Nursing (AACN) published a comprehensive list of nursing competencies under 10 domains.
- The consensus model defines APRN practice, describes the APRN regulatory model, identifies the titles to be used, defines specialty, and describes the emergence of new roles and population foci.
- Each state and territory establishes levels of supervision for APRNs. Supervision is described as one health care professional overseeing another's practice.
- Ethics define a clear set of rules commonly accepted and followed and can direct the creation of policies and procedures.

ACTIVITIES

Compare and Contrast States' Scope of Practice

- Students (individually or in groups) will be assigned two or more states with varying levels of practice authority and asked to compare and contrast each state's scope of practice.
- Consider either a discussion board posting or a live, interactive student discussion during class time.

Discuss Health Care Ethics

- Students (individuals or groups) will be given ethical situations to consider.
- Students are to create and post 1–3-minute videos explaining the situation, their resolution, and the guiding ethical principles.

Annotated Bibliography

- Students must find and read five peer-reviewed journal articles on aspects of APRN practice (legal, ethical, licensure, scope of practice, etc.).
- Students will create an annotated bibliography based on the five articles.
- Students will verbally report their findings to the class.

REFERENCES

American Association of Nurse Practitioners. (2022). *State practice environment.* https://www.aanp.org/advocacy/state/state-practice-environment

American Nurses Association. (2015). *Code of ethics for nurses with interpretive statements.* https://www.nursingworld.org/practice-policy/nursing-excellence/ethics/code-of-ethics-for-nurses/

Benedict, S., & Kuhla, J. (1999). Nurses' participation in the euthanasia programs of Nazi Germany. *Western Journal of Nursing Research, 21*(2), 127–274. doi.org/10.1177/01939459922043749

Brenan, M. (2023). Nurses retain top ethics rating in U.S., but below 2020 high. *Gallup.* https://news.gallup.com/poll/467804/nurses-retain-top-ethics-rating-below-2020-high.aspx

Haddad, L. M., & Geiger, R. A. (2022). *Nursing ethical considerations.* StatPearls. https://www.ncbi.nlm.nih.gov/books/NBK526054/

Motacki, K., & Burke, K. M. (2017). *Nursing delegation and management of patient care* (2nd ed.). Elsevier.

Peacock, M., & Hernandez, S. (2020). A concept analysis of nurse practitioner autonomy. *Journal of the American Association of Nurse Practitioners, 32*(2), 113–119. https://doi.org/10.1097/JXX.0000000000000374

Peterson, P. A., Keller, T., Way, S. M. & Borges, W. J. (2015). Autonomy and empowerment in advanced practice registered nurses: Lessons from New Mexico. *Journal of the American Association of Nurse Practitioners, 27,* 363–370. https://doi.org/10.1002/2327-6924.12202

Poghosyan, L., Ghaffari, A., Liu, J., Jin, H., & Martsolf, G. (2020). State policy change and organizational response: Expansion of nurse practitioner scope of practice regulations in New York state. *Nursing Outlook, 69*, 74–83. doi.org/10.1016/j.outlook.2020.08.007

Poghosyan, L., Stein, J. H., Liu, J., Spetz, J., Osakwe, Z. T., & Martsolf, G. (2022). State-level scope of practice regulations for nurse practitioners impact work environments: Six state investigation. *Research in Health and Nursing, 45*, 516–524. https://doi.org/10.1002/nur.22253

Ritter, A. Z., Bowles, K. H., O'Sullivan, A. L., Carthon, M. B., & Fairman, J. A. (2018). A policy analysis of legally required supervision of nurse practitioners and other health professionals. *Nursing Outlook, 66*, 551–559. doi.org/10.1016/j.outlook.2018.05.004

Taylor, L. N., & Gilchrist, S. (2020). How state scope of practice policies impact NP care. *American Journal of Nursing, 120*(9), 21–22.

CHAPTER 10

Transitioning From Registered Nurse to Advanced Practice Nurse/Nurse Practitioner

Carole Mackavey and Tammy Stout

OBJECTIVES

Upon completion of the chapter, the student will be able to

1. explain the importance of a transition to a practice program
2. discuss the importance of excellent communication skills
3. demonstrate skills for participating in crucial conversation
4. describe the role of the advanced practice nurse in the medical team

QUESTIONS/CHALLENGES

1. What obstacles do you anticipate when transitioning from student APRN to practicing APRN?
2. How will you explain the role of the APRN to a new medical team?

INTRODUCTION

The transition from registered nurse to advanced practice nurse (APN) is a dynamic process that occurs over time (Mackavey & Brykczynski, 2022). APNs demonstrate academic competency when they graduate and pass the National Nurse Practitioner exam, proctored by the American Association of Nurse Practitioners (AANP) or the American Association of Colleges of Nursing (AACN). APNs graduate with increased knowledge and skills from previous experience or through the program's clinical rotation, expanded autonomy, and decision-making.

The number of nurse practitioners (NPs) in the United States is steadily increasing, although the shortage of advanced practice providers (APPs) remains. The American Association of Nurse Practitioners (AANP) reports there are currently over 355,000 NPs licensed in the United States (AANP National Nurse Practitioner Database, 2023). APPs are highly trained and specialized in health care (Dillon et al., 2016). Nationwide, NPs are working in intensive care units (ICUs) at a much higher frequency due to increased demand, resident work-hour restrictions, and an overall increase in the acuity of patients admitted to tertiary medical centers (Typpo et al., 2012; Moote et al., 2011). Results of multiple studies indicate that NPs provide safe and effective care comparable in quality to their physician colleagues (Typpo et al., 2012; Kleinpell et al., 2015).

Most new NPs have only worked for approximately 2 years before pursuing an advanced degree. Although they are seasoned nurses well versed in coordinating care for patients, families, and valued members of the health care team, transitioning from the registered nurse (RN) role to that of an advanced practice registered nurse (APRN) can be a difficult and highly stressful time for a new graduate (Barnes, 2015; Hart & Bowen, 2016). The new graduate's journey from RN to APN is often filled with feelings of anxiety and stress (Stiner et al., 2008). New NPs report feeling overwhelmed, vulnerable, and inadequate while navigating the role of the APN. Poronsky (2013) noted that the transition of the novice NP to expert was "anxiety, role confusion, stress, insecurity, self-doubt, apprehension, emotional turmoil, and isolation." Transitioning from "expert" RN to "novice" NP (Benner, 1984) has been reportedly associated with expressions of inadequacies and vulnerabilities by NPs.

Brown and Olshansky (1998) identified four role transition stages for new NPs:

1. **laying the foundation:** The new NP begins to prepare for the certification examination and securing licensure, finding employment while leaving academia behind.
2. **launching:** Initial employment is secured, and the "first year" of practice begins. The novice NP learns to navigate the work environment while confronting his/her feelings of inadequacy.
3. **meeting the challenge:** The NP begins to feel a sense of belonging and competency in the clinical site.
4. **broadening the perspective:** New responsibilities are taken on and, in fact, sought out by the NP (Brown & Olshansky, 1998; Hill & Sawatzky, 2011).

Many employers expect the new NP graduate to care for the same number of patients as an experienced provider. Nevertheless, more time is typically required by the novice NP to examine patients, document, review charts, investigate laboratory values, review treatment plans, and learn how to accomplish simple and complex tasks. These additional stressors can lead to workplace dissatisfaction, thus adversely affecting overall APN retention. Hill and Sawatzky (2011) recommend creating a partnership or mentorship between novice NPs and experienced APNs. The mentor would be able to provide emotional support and aid in organizational integration during the transition period.

"Leaving the comfort zone of being an experienced RN for a new career as an inexperienced advanced practice registered nurse (APRN) is one of the greatest difficulties of the APRN transition to practice" (Urbanowicz, 2019, p. 1). New APRNs resoundingly express a lack of self-confidence as they begin their new practitioner roles. Career adjustment periods can impact APRNs' development and decision on whether to remain in nursing (Hoff et al., 2019). Hart and Bowen (2016) further assessed new NPs' perceptions of their preparation for transition into practice in a post-academic setting. They found that 62.6% of respondents agreed or strongly agreed to adequate clinical support in their first year of practice. Only 42.2% of respondents described feeling well or generally prepared after graduation. Most participants, a total of 58%, expressed extreme interest in a postgraduate residency program. Of the 50% who provided written feedback, 90% expressed needing a postgraduate formal mentor or residency.

Residency and fellowship programs for new graduate NPs have been supported by the National Nurse Practitioner Residency Training Consortium to assist health care organizations in establishing training programs (Martsolf et al., 2017). These residency programs are a relatively new practice and need more standardization in structure. The programs vary widely by specialty focus, type of organization overseeing the program, and length of the program.

In addition, orientation programs have been implemented to create a smoother transition into the new graduate NP's practice. St-Martin and colleagues (2015) showed that preceptorship experience strongly impacted the new APRN's development. Thus, preceptors willing to teach and provide feedback to the new NPs offered positive mentoring. Residency programs cannot be implemented without motivated, trained, and compensated preceptors (Bush, 2014).

The Institute of Medicine's (IOM, 2010) *The Future of Nursing* report noted that to meet patients' needs in the future, academic institutions must train more NPs to meet growing levels of clinical sophistication. Transition-to-practice (TTP) programs for advanced practice nurses (APNs) and physician assistants (PAs) have been available since the 1970s (Kesten et al., 2019). The IOM report further recommended residency programs for NPs after completing an advanced practice degree program (IOM, 2010). However, to date, very few formal residency programs for NPs exist. These residency programs are a relatively new practice and lack standardization in structure. They vary widely by specialty focus, type of organization overseeing the program, and program length.

In January 2019, the Commission on College Nursing Education (CCNE) released a statement, forming the Nurse Practitioner Residency/Fellowship Standards Committee to create accreditation standards to help guide academic nursing residency programs nationwide. The CCNE requires 500 hours of clinical training before graduating with an advanced practice degree (CCNE, 2019). However, requirements are currently being reviewed for increased hours required for accreditation (CCNE, 2023). Residency and fellowship programs for new graduate NPs are supported by the National Nurse Practitioner Residency Training Consortium to assist health care organizations in establishing training programs (Martsolf et al., 2017). Brown and colleagues (2015) highlighted five "must-haves" for building a framework for a residency program or characteristics of a successful resident: interprofessional training, a leadership or policy component, quality improvement and scholarship, diagnostic skill honing and special skill readiness, and dedicated mentorship and role development.

In July 2017, the Cleveland Clinic launched the APRN and physician assistance (PA) onboarding program, modeled after the

Accreditation Council for Graduate Education (ACGME), American Nurses Credentialing Center (ANCC), and Accreditation and Review Commission on Physician Assistant Education (ARC-PA) accreditation. Within this program, new hires gradually increased autonomous practice after 3 months of employment and continued nonclinical training within the group overall. During the second 6 months, nonclinical training was reduced. Orientation programs have also been implemented to create a smoother transition into the new graduate NP's practice. St-Martin and colleagues (2015) showed that preceptorship experience strongly impacted the new APRN's development. Preceptors willing to teach and provide feedback to the new NP provided positive mentoring (Bush, 2014). In 2016, the ANCC published the Practice Transition Accreditation Program (PTAP) to develop criteria and guidelines for organizations establishing residency or fellowship programs. To date, 440 sites have one or more programs accredited by the ANCC (2023).

It is unclear why formal APRN transition opportunities are not more common, but a lack of willing preceptors is one hypothesized causation. A 2018 national report by an NP recruitment firm, NP NOW, predicted the number of NPs practicing throughout the United States would fall to 29,400 by 2025 (NPNow.com, 2019). In 2019, Indeed.com reported that 59.7% of NP jobs were in the top 15 most difficult to fill. Turnover rates for NPs were reportedly twice that of physician colleagues (NP.com, 2019; Barnes, 2015; Faraz, 2016). NP fellowship/residency programs have been established in all 50 states and Washington, DC. Thirty-two states and Washington, DC have full-practice privileges (AANP, 2023). Nurses engaged in advanced practice have expanded autonomy, skill, and decision-making levels (Gardner et al., 2007; Manning & Neville, 2009). Many other states have full practice authority bills currently proposed pending legislative decisions. Advanced practice nurses must complete 500 to 1,500 clinical hours, while physicians must complete 6,000 hours (MidlevelU, 2017). This variation could leave transitioning the APRN practice with little opportunity for the new NP to gain confidence and experience. Annual costs per APRN trainee are estimated at as much as $100,000, with two-thirds of expenses supporting the cost of the new APRN (Hoff et al., 2019). In addition, Hart and Bowen (2016) reported new NPs being the least prepared for billing and coding, simple office procedures, electrocardiogram and radiology interpretation, microscopy, and mental illness management, thus being susceptible to a lack of reimbursement:

> Although these studies can be considered in the development of a transition program, to date, there is little to no literature related to how transition programs might be received or how a program would impact the outcomes of length of employment, job satisfaction, confidence to practice, ability to perform, or the impact a new APRN may have on patient care. (Urbanowicz, 2019, p. 52)

ROLE TRANSITION

Role transition begins with the educational program. The transition process is stressful and often influenced by personal factors. APRNs are encouraged to think critically, synthesize the information presented, and demonstrate increased skills. Realistic expectations are critical to reducing stress. There will be doubt, and students often question their identity. The imposter phenomenon, or feeling like a fake or you "don't belong," is also very common and should not be thought of as abnormal. Throughout the program, the student will begin to develop competency, gain confidence, experience the beginning of the role change, and develop a support network of fellow students and faculty. Some of the factors present in role transitions include one's own personal associations with the transition; planning or anticipating the change; having adequate support systems, possessing the proper knowledge, skills, and attitudes from school; and, finally, the expectations usually linked to faculty mentors and preceptors.

Barnes et al. (2022) examined the factors that impacted the new nurse practitioner role transition and developed a scale to measure the role transition. The five factors were identified as two intrinsic—a sense of purpose, perceived competence, and/or self-confidence—and three extrinsic concepts—compensation, organizational alignment, and mentorship (Barnes et al., 2020).

Uncertainty is a primary concern with new APNs; clinical decision-making is stressful. The New AACN Competency-Based Essential provides an opportunity for each clinical and diagnostic reasoning to ease the burden of uncertainty. Uncertainty will always be a challenge. Doubting oneself is frequently a challenge. Something important to remember is increasing evidence that shows NPs provide quality care equal to or better than, in some cases, their physician counterparts (Buerhaus, 2018).

There has been considerable research on the APN role transition over the years. The same themes continue to emerge, building a solid framework for nursing practice that supports evidence-based practice research and strong collaboration, direct patient-centered care through strong communication skills, a thorough history, and physical and critical thinking. The final component is professionalism through demonstrated leadership, self-reflection, communication, and lifelong learning. The role of the APN continues to evolve and grow as states fight for independent practice, and the role is recognized in other countries.

COMMUNICATION: DIFFICULT CONVERSATIONS

APNs often develop a strong rapport with their patients. Straightforward, honest communication can enhance the relationship.

Difficult conversations are uncomfortable. APNs are responsible for delivering bad news, calming upset patients, and providing patient education by explaining the treatment plans and insurance requirements. Very often, sitting down at eye level with patients and calmly explaining their situation facilitates the best response. The goal of the APN is to create a positive outcome. Unfortunately, it is not always possible. Some potentially difficult patient situations include the following:

- consulting "Dr. Google" (three clicks to cancer)
- failure to accept the diagnosis
- lack of trust related to no diagnosis, despite having signs and symptoms
- noncompliance
- a negative focus on continuing symptoms, as opposed to recognizing progress (Mosher, 2022)

Several techniques can be used when having a difficult conversation. The first is to provide honest, direct, and respectful feedback. Use a communication technique that encourages open dialogue. Make sure you are well informed. Finally, keep communication lines open. Consider the example in which an APN must inform a 68-year-old female patient that her mammogram is positive for invasive breast cancer. The APN sits down with the patient and explains the findings. The patient is reticent. The APN also tells her that she has arranged for the patient to have the biopsy for staging with the breast surgeon and an appointment with the oncologist to determine a care plan. She is free to cancel the appointment and make her own. Before departing, the APN asks if she has any questions. A follow-up call was completed about a week later, and a message was left for the patient. The patient returned to the clinic smiling and hugging the APN, thanking her for her foresight and help. Sometimes, the patient is overwhelmed by the diagnosis; having a plan can help ease the burden.

> "As we navigate through 2023, we will face more complex and difficult conversations with our family, friends, and colleagues. We'll be challenged to truly listen, communicate with respect and empathy, and hold space for hard conversations." (Management Executive Education, 2023)

FUNCTIONING AS A MEMBER OF THE HEALTH CARE TEAM

Strengthening health care systems is challenging, and the most promising solutions can be found in interprofessional collaboration (WHO, 2010). Role clarity between providers is crucial in a smooth functioning team (Ulrich & Crider, 2017). Gysin et al. (2019) identified that general physicians in the United States and other countries lack knowledge regarding the APN role (Gysin, 2019).

A study by Chen et al. (2012) found that good communication, job satisfaction, and work environment positively influence teamwork (Chen et al., 2012). Kilpatrick et al. (2020) conducted a systematic review to evaluate interventions to improve health care team functioning. They found that brief interventions effectively clarified the roles of the health care team and improved team functioning (Kilpatrick et al., 2020). High-fidelity simulation, structured communication and speaking up, and leadership training showed promise. Interprofessional education can provide learners with a better understanding of their roles and aid in developing effective collaborative practice.

PATIENT-CENTERED CARE

Person-centered care is a key focus of the new AACN competencies to achieve better health outcomes. The Affordable Care Act

(ACA) increased the number of people with health insurance, increasing the population of patients receiving primary care as a result. This increased need for primary care providers has added to the pressure felt by the new APN.

A vast number of Baby Boomers are close approaching retirement age. There is an increase in patient complexity, and many patients are presenting with multiple chronic diseases. Electronic health records, insufficient support staff, and public demand for competency are complicating the entry to practice.

Fortunately well-established principles for patient or person-centered care are readily available to practitioners. The Picker Institute's eight principles were identified and established in 1993 and are still discussed today.

The Eight Picker Principles of Patient-Centered Care

- respect for patient's values, preferences, and expressed needs
- coordination and integration of care
- information, communication, and education
- physical comfort
- emotional support and alleviation of fear and anxiety
- involvement of family and friends
- continuity and transition
- access to care

For more on Picker Principles, visit the following web page: https://picker.org/who-we-are/the-picker-principles-of-person-centred-care/.

In Buerhaus's (2018) report, APNs can potentially help solve the problem of Americans' access to quality primary care. APNs are more likely to practice in rural and underserved areas, where access to primary care is a key issue. APRNs provide quality health care, and working with physicians collaboratively can meet community health care needs (Buerhaus, 2018).

CHAPTER SUMMARY

The Future of Nursing 2020–2030 committee identifies nurses' well-being as essential to delivering high-quality patient care (National Academy of Medicine, 2020). Thus, there is a critical need to understand novice NPs' transition to practice (Barnes et al., 2021). The increasing complexity of our health care system, the increased provider workloads, and the risk to one's health associated with pandemics make it essential for the employer and new NP to create a smooth and supportive transition period. Open communication and strong mentorship during orientation are necessary to ease the stress associated with role transition.

Food for Thought

What do you anticipate will be your biggest challenge transitioning from RN to APN, and how would you address the issues?

KEY POINTS

- Straightforward, honest communication can enhance the relationship.
- APRNs are an integral part of the health care team.
- Evidence-based practice and strong collaboration is critical to advanced nursing practice.
- Role clarity between providers is crucial in a smooth functioning team.

ACTIVITIES

1. Reflect on what you anticipate to be the most challenging part of transition practice. How would you explain the role of the NP to other health care team members?
2. After watching this brief video, "Crucial Conversations" (https://www.youtube.com/watch?v=ryCeARRE-KA), practice the listed role-play scenarios. You are also encouraged to watch the following videos as helpful role-play examples: "How Do I Handle Someone Being Defensive?" (https://www.youtube.com/watch?v=mBouwZM0qqU) and "Giving Constructive Feedback to a Co-Worker—Role Play" (https://www.youtube.com/watch?v=80chgXavudM).
   a. Role-play participating in a difficult conversation.
   b. Critique a difficult conversation.

REFERENCES

American Association of Nurse Practitioners. (2017). *National nurse practitioner database*. https://www.aanp.org/about/all-about-nps/np-fact-sheet

American Nurses Credentialing Center. (AACN). (2023).

Barnes, H. (2015). Exploring the factors that influence nurse practitioner role transition. *The Journal for Nurse Practitioners.*, *11*(2), 178–183.

Barnes, H., Faraz Covelli, A., & Rubright, J. D. (2021). Development of the novice nurse practitioner role transition scale: An exploratory factor analysis. *Journal of the American Association of Nurse Practitioners*, *34*(1), 79–88. https://doi.org/10.1097/JXX.0000000000000566

Benner, P. (1984). *From novice to expert: Excellence and power in clinical nursing practice*. Addison-Wesley.

Brown, M. A., & Olshansky, E. F. (1997). From limbo to legitimacy: A theoretical model of the transition to the primary care nurse practitioner role. *Nursing Research*, *46*(1), 46–51.

Brown, K., Poppe, A., Kaminetzky, C., Wipf, J., & Woods, N. F. (2015). Recommendations for nurse practitioner residency programs. *Nurse Educator, 40*(3), 148–151. https://doi.org/10.1097/NNE.0000000000000117

Buerhaus, P. (2018, September 18). *Nurse practitioners: A solution to America's primary care crisis.* American Enterprise Institute. https://www.aei.org/research-products/report/nurse-practitioners-a-solution-to-americas-primary-care-crisis/

Bush, C. (2014). Postgraduate nurse practitioner training: What nurse executives need to know. *Journal of Nursing Administration, 14*(12), 625–627.

Carthon, J. M. B., Brom, H., Poghosyan, L., Daus, M., Todd, B., & Aiken, L. (2020). Supportive clinical practice environments associated with patient-centered care. *The Journal for Nurse Practitioners: JNP, 16*(4), 294–298. https://doi.org/10.1016/j.nurpra.2020.01.019

Castellucci, M. (2016). Medical schools tackle primary care shortage. *Modern Health Care.* www.modernhealthcare.com/article/20161105/MAGAZINE/311059982/medical-schools-tackle-primary-care-shortages.

Chien, S. F., Wan, T. T., & Chen, Y. C. (2012). Factors influencing teamwork and collaboration within a tertiary medical center. *World Journal of Methodology, 2*(2), 18–23. https://doi.org/10.5662/wjm.v2.i2.18

Dillon, D., Dolansky, M, Casey, K., & Kelley, C. (2016). Factors related to successful transition to practice for acute care nurse practitioners. *AACM Advanced Critical Care, 27*(2), 173–182. https://doi.org/10.4037/aacnacc2016619

Gardner, G., Chang, A., & Duffield, C. (2007). Making nursing work: Breaking through the role confusion of advanced practice nursing. *Journal of Advanced Nursing, 57*, 382–391.

Gysin, S., Sottas, B., Odermatt, M., & Essig, S. (2019). Advanced practice nurses' and general practitioners' first experiences with introducing the advanced practice nurse role to Swiss primary care: A qualitative study. *BMC Family Practice, 20*(1), 163. https://doi.org/10.1186/s12875-019-1055-z

Hart, A. M., & Bowen, A. (2016). New nurse practitioners' perceptions of preparedness for and transition into practice. *The Journal for Nurse Practitioners. 8*(12), 545–552. https://doi.org/10.1016/j.nurpra.2016.04.018

Hill, L. & Sawatzky, J. (2011). Transitioning into the nurse practitioner role through mentorship. *Journal of Professional Nursing, 27*(3), 161–167.

Hoff, T., Carabetta, S., Collinson, G. E. (2019). Satisfaction, burnout, and turnover among nurse practitioners and physician assistants: A review of the empirical literature. *Medical Care Research and Review.*, *76*(1), 3–31.

Institute of Medicine (IOM). (2010). *The future of nursing: Leading change, advancing health.* The National Academic Press.

Kilpatrick, K., Paquette, L., Jabbour, M., Tchouaket, E., Fernandez, N., Al Hakim, G., Landry, V., Gauthier, N., Beaulieu, M.-D., & Dubois, C.-A. (2020). Systematic review of the characteristics of brief team interventions to clarify roles and improve functioning in health care teams. *PloS One*, *15*(6), e0234416–e0234416. https://doi.org/10.1371/journal.pone.0234416

Kleinpell R., Ward, N. S., Kelso, L. A., Mollenkopf, F. P., Jr., & Houghton, D. (2015). Provider to patient ratios for nurse practitioners and physician assistants in critical care units. *American Journal of Critical Care*, *24*(3), e16–e21.

Mackavey, C. & Bryczykski (2022). Role development in the advanced practice nurse. In Mary Fran Tracy, Eileen T. O'Grady, Susanne J. Phillips (Eds.), *Hamric and Hanson's advanced practice nursing: An integrative approach* (7th ed.). Elsevier.

Management Executive Education. (2023). *Navigating difficult conversations in 2023.* https://exec.mit.edu/s/blog-post/navigating-difficult-conversations-in-2023-MCQDH3AMA36JGHDEXRS2T2HLPDIM)

Manning, L., & Neville, S. (2009). Work-role transition: From staff nurse to clinical nurse educator. *Nursing Praxis in New Zealand*, *25*, 41–53.

Martsolf, G., PhuongGiang, N., Freund, D., & Poghosyan, L. (2017). What we know about postgraduate nurse practitioner residency and fellowship programs. *The Journal for Nurse Practitioners*, *13*(7), 482–487.

McGuier, E. A., Kolko, D. J., Klem, M. L., Feldman, J., Kinkler, G., Diabes, M. A., Weingart, L. R., & Wolk, C. B. (2021). Team functioning and implementation of innovations in healthcare and human service settings: a systematic review protocol. *Systematic Reviews*, *10*(1), 189. https://doi.org/10.1186/s13643-021-01747-w

Merriam-Webster. (n.d.). Communication. In *Merriam-Webster.com dictionary.* https://www.merriam-webster.com/dictionary/communication

MidlevelU. (2017). *MD vs. NP vs. PA: Here's how the number of clinical hours compare.* www.midlevelu.com/blog/md-vs-np-vs-pa-heres-how-number-clinical-hours-compare.

Moote, M., Krsek, C., Kleinpell, R., Todd, B. (2011). Physician assistant and nurse practitioner utilization in academic medical centers. *American Journal of Medical Quality, 26*(6), 452–460.

Mosher, A. (2022). How NPs can tackle difficult conversations with patients and families. *Nurse Practitioner Online.* https://www.nursepractitioneronline.com/articles/how-to-tackle-difficult-conversations/

Picker Institute's eight principles of person-centered care. https://nexusipe.org/informing/resource-center/picker-institute%E2%80%99s-eight-principles-person-centered-care

Poronsky, C. B. (2013). Exploring the transition from registered nurse to family nurse practitioner. *Journal of Professional Nursing, 29*(6), 350–358.

Steiner, S. H., McLaughlin, D. G., Hyde, R. S., Brown, R. H., & Burman, M. E. (2008). Role transition during rn-tofnp education. *Journal of Nursing Education, 47*(10), 441–447. https://doi.org/10.3928/01484834-20081001-07

St-Martin, L., Harripaul, A., Antonacci, R., Laframboise, D., & Purden, M. (2015). Advanced beginner to competent practitioner: new graduate nurses' perceptions of strategies that facilitate or hinder development. *Journal of Continuing Education in Nursing, 46*(9), 392–400.

Typpo, K. V., Tcharmtchi, M. H., Thomas, E. J., Kelly, P. A., Castillo, L. D., Singh, H. (2012). Impact of resident duty hour limits on safety in the ICU: A national survey of pediatric and neonatal intensivists. *Pediatric Critical Care Medicine, 13*(5):578–582.

Ulrich, B., & Crider, N. M. (2017). Using teams to improve outcomes and performance. *Nephrology Nursing Journal J, 44,* 141–151. PMID: 29165965

Urbanowicz, J. (2019). APRN transition to practice: Program development tips. *The Nurse Practitioner, 44*(12), 50–55. https://doi.org/10.1097/01.npr.0000605520.88939.d1

World Health Organization [WHO]. (2010). Framework for Action on interprofessional education & collaborative practice. World Health Organization protocol. *Systematic Reviews, 10*(1), 189–189. https://doi.org/10.1186/s13643-021-01747-w

INDEX

A

access in telehealth, 127
accountable care organizations (ACOs), 180
Accreditation and Review Commission on Physician Assistant Education (ARC-PA), 220
Accreditation Council for Graduate Education (ACGME), 220
adult learning theory, 74–75
advanced practice nurses (APNs), 215–227
  Canada, 14–15
  China, 15–16
  clinical role of, 33–34
  DNP-prepared, 32
  doctoral education, 31–32
  entry-level degrees for, 30
  Netherlands, 16–17
  primary specializations, 34
advanced practice nursing (APN)
  caring for vulnerable populations, 113–114
  COVID-19 pandemic, 7–10
  education pathway, 29–41
  history, 2–12
  international practice, 12–20
  nurse practitioners, 5
  nursing response to a crisis, 5–6
  overview, 2
  practice, 131
  resistance against, 3–5
  simulation in, 59–97
advanced practice nursing education, 94–95
advanced practice nursing programs, 69–71
advanced practice providers (APPs), 10, 216
advanced practice registered nurses (APRNs), 5, 33, 104, 162, 183, 198–200, 218
  characteristics of, 142
  Consensus Model, 38
  domains, 202–204
  in leadership and project management, 141–158
  leading teams, 145–146
  leveraging influence, 145–146
  organizational culture, 143–145
  primary specializations, 34
advanced registered nurse practitioner (ARNP), 5
Affordable Care Act (ACA), 7, 162, 164, 171–175, 224–225
American Academy of Nursing's Edge Runners initiative, 113
American Association of Colleges of Nursing (AACN), 5, 30, 49, 68–69, 82, 95, 142, 201, 216
  competencies in APN education and role, 47–55
  Essentials, 35
American Association of Nurse Practitioners (AANP), 5, 199, 205–206, 216
American Data Privacy and Protection Act (ADPPA), 165
American Medical Association, 172
American Nurses Association (ANA), 36, 208
American Nurses Association's (ANA) Code of Ethics, 148–149
American Nurses Credentialing Center (ANCC), 220
American Rescue Plan Act, 164
APRN Scope of Practice (SOP), 199
artificial intelligence (AI), 124
assessment via telehealth, 127

associate degrees in nursing (ADN), 68
Association of American Medical Colleges (AAMC), 127
Association of SP Educators Standards of Best Practice, 82
asynchronous telehealth, 126
Atlantic Red Cross, 5
audio telehealth, 132
augmented reality (AR), 124
Australia
  as developed high income country, 171
  NPs, 13–14
Australian College of Nurse Practitioners, 13

B

bachelors of science in nursing (BSN), 68
Bandura, Albert, 75
Barnes, H., 222
Berg, J. A., 3
Bloom's revised taxonomy, 75
boards of nursing (BON), 198–199
Boswell, C., 32
Bowen, A., 218, 221
briefing, 63
  and prebriefing, 86–87
Brown, K., 219
Brown, M. A., 217
Buerhaus, P., 225

C

Canada
  APNs, 14–15
  clinical nurse specialists, 14
  NPs, 14–15
ceiling preemption, 169
Center for Medicare and Medicaid Innovation (CMS Innovation Center), 178
Centers for Medicare and Medicaid Services (CMS), 131–132, 134, 161, 181
certified nurse-midwives (CNM), 37
Certified Registered Nurse Anesthetists (CRNAs), 10–11, 39–40
Chase, Martha Jenkins, 64
Chen, Y. C., 224
child immunization, 166
Children's Health Insurance Program (CHIP), 164
Children's Online Privacy Protection Act (COPPA), 131
China
  APNs, 15–16
  Sichuan Provincial People's Hospital (SPPH), 16
clinical hours, 200
clinical leadership, 142
clinical microsystem, 143
clinical nurse specialists (CNSs), 37–39
  and COVID-19 pandemic, 39
clinical reasoning, 53–54
Clinton, Bill, 164
cognitive bias, 54
Commission on College Nursing Education (CCNE), 219
communication, 62
  Crew Resource Management Principles, 62
  transition from registered nurse to advanced practice nurse, 222–224
  via telehealth, 127
competency
  AACN, in APN education and role, 47–55
  -based clinical education, 53–54
  in education and practice, 48
  telehealth, 127–128
competency-based education (CBE), 48–54
  competency-based clinical education, 53–54
  domains of competence, 49–50
Congressional Budget Office (CBO), 179
consensus model, 204–205
Consolidated Appropriations Act of 2023, 130
Consolidated Omnibus Budget Reconciliation Act (COBRA), 164
continued professional development, 72–73
continuing education (CE), 200–201

Coronavirus Aid, Relief, and Economic Security Act (CARES Act), 183
COVID-19 pandemic, 6, 20–21, 76, 94–95, 123, 128, 132
 advanced practice nursing, 7–10
 and clinical nurse specialists (CNSs), 39
 Canadian health care system, 14
 certified registered nurse anesthetists, 10–11
 health policy and, 181–184
 impact on NP education, 40–41
 nursing educators, 35
 political issues, 169
Crew Resource Management Principles, 62–63
 briefing, 62
 communication, 62
 debriefing, 63
 decision-making, 63
 leadership, 62
 mutual monitoring, 63
 team adaptability, 63
critical thinking, 48

D

data collection via telehealth, 127
debriefing, 63
 analysis, 90
 as simulation phase, 89–92
 conducted within a group, 89
 effective, 90
 methods, 90–92
 post-simulation, 90
 reaction, 90
 self-led, 89
 summary, 91
Debriefing Assessment for Simulation in Health Care (DASH) tool, 92
decision making, 63
deliberate practice theory, 75
delivery performance, 152–153, 155
demonstration rooms, 64
DeNicola, N., 129
Department of Health and Human Services (DHHS), 7
design/designing
 as simulation phases, 89
 simulation, 84–86
development approach, PM, 151, 155
disproportionate share hospital (DSH), 180–181
doctor of nursing practice (DNP), 30, 200
 challenges faced by, 32
 degree, 31
 nurse executive, 35–36
 -prepared APN practitioner, 32
Donnelly, S., 18
Ducey, Douglas A., 169

E

educational simulations, 67
effective team leader, 145
the Emergency Food Assistance Program (TEFAP), 182
Emergency Medical Treatment and Labor Act (EMTALA), 164
emergency use authorizations (EUA), 183
equity in telehealth, 127
Essentials: Core Competencies for Professional Nursing Education, 30, 68–69, 95, 142
ethical practices and legal requirements for telehealth, 128
ethics, defind, 208
evaluation
 formative, 92–93
 high-stakes, 93–94
 in simulation, 92–94
 summative, 93
evaluation tools, 94
eVisits, 132
experiential learning cycle, 96
experiential learning theory, 73–74

F

Fair Credit Reporting Act, 165
Families First Coronavirus Act, 164
Families First Coronavirus Response Act, 182
Family Educational Rights and Privacy Act, 165
Federal Drug Administration (FDA), 167
federal poverty level (FPL), 173
Federal Trade Commission (FTC), 167

fee-for-service (FFS) rates, 179–180
Ford, Lorretta, 2–4
formative evaluation, 92–93
full practice authority (FPA), 8–9, 205–206
Future of Nursing, 8
Future of Nursing: Leading Change and Advancing Health (Institute of Medicine), 141
Future of Nursing Report, 2010, 32

G

Gaba, D. M., 60
Geiger, R. A., 208
graduate degree, 200
Graham, A. C., 70
Gramm-Leach-Bliley Act, 165
Grenny, J., 145
Guidelines on Advanced Practice Nursing, 12
Gysin, S., 224

H

Haddad, L. M., 208
Harrington, Michael, 2
Hart, A. M., 218, 221
Hart, Brad, 169
health care, 110–111
Health Care Simulation Standards of Best Practice (HSSOBP) guidelines, 82, 85–87
health disparity, 108–109
  and Healthy People 2020, 108
  defined, 108
  vs. health equity, 108–113
Health Education England (HEE), 18–19
health equity, 110–113
  defined, 110
  health disparity *vs.*, 108–113
Health Information Technology for Economic and Clinical Health Act, 166
Health Information Technology for Economic and Clinical Health (HITECH), 131
health insurance
  cost, 175
  cost of living/care, 175
  geographical areas, 175
  individual *vs.* family enrollment, 175
  obtaining and renewing, 174–175
  older adults, 175
  tobacco users, 175
  variations, 175
Health Insurance Portability and Accountability Act (HIPAA), 131, 163, 165–166
health policy
  access to health care, 171–173
  advocacy and, 161–188
  advocating for change, 170–171
  consumer protection provisions, 173–174
  cost-containment, 179–180
  COVID-19 pandemic and, 181–184
  defined, 162–163
  funding, cost containment measures, and impact on health care costs, 178–179
  impact on health care, 164–170
  Medicaid, 180–181
  Medicare, 179–180
  obtaining and renewing health insurance, 174–175
  overview, 161–162
  policy change, 163–164
  post-introduction analysis, 176–181
  transparency, 175–176
health policy leadership, 142
Healthy People 2020, 108
high-fidelity manikins, 80
high-quality simulations, 72
high-stakes evaluation, 92–94
Hill-Burton Act, 65
Hill, L., 217
HIPAA Enforcement Rule, 166
human papillomavirus (HPV), 177

I

ICN Nurse Practitioner/Advanced Practice Network (ICN NP/APNN), 13
influencers, 145
informatics and health care technologies, 203–204
Institute of Medicine (IOM), 31, 122–123

intensive care units (ICUs), 216
International Council of Nurses (ICN), 12, 17
International Nursing Association of Clinical Simulation and Learning (INASCL), 60, 65, 85, 89
  Standards Committee, 87, 89
  standards of best practice for evaluation of learning and performance, 93
  standards of best practice for simulation, 95
interprofessional partnerships, 203
Irish Nurses and Midwives Organisation (INMO), 18

J

Jefferies Simulation Model, 85
Johnson, Lyndon B., 2

K

Kiley, Deborah, 3–4
Kilpatrick, K., 224
King-Dailey, K., 128
Knopp, A., 70
knowledge for nursing practice, 202
Knowles, Malcolm, 74–75
Kolb, David Allen, 73–74, 89, 96

L

Laerdal, 65
leadership, 62
  authentic, 39
  bidirectional, 143
  clinical, 142
  executive, 31, 35
  health policy, 142
  nurse executive, 35–36
  professional, 142
  systems, 142
legal parameters of care and practice, 197–213
  consensus model, 204–205
  health care, law, and ethics, 208–211
  overview, 198
  practice act, 198–204
  United States, levels of supervision, 205–208
licensure and credentialing, 131
life cycle performance, 151, 155
Lioce, L., 60
low-fidelity manikins, 80
Lynch, Judith, 3–4

M

Madam du Courdray, 63
manikins, 80
master advanced nursing practice (MANP), 16
master of science in nursing (MSN), 200
McArthur, Donna B., 4
Meadows, Richard, 4
measurement performance, 153–155
Medicaid, 2, 131, 162, 164, 168, 172–173, 180–181
medical education, 129
Medical Education Technologies, Inc. (METI), 65
medical loss ratio (MLR), 180
Medicare, 2, 11, 132, 134–135, 162, 172–173, 179–180
Menkiena, C., 37
mental health
  impacts of SDOHs on, 114–115
  outcomes, 114–115
  strained, 11–12
Merit-based Incentive Payment System (MIPS), 182
Miller, George, 75
mobile health (mHealth), 126
mutual monitoring, 63

N

National Aeronautics and Space Administration (NASA), 62
national certification, 200
National Council of State Boards of Nursing (NCSBN), 68, 201
National Disaster Medical System, 183
National League of Nursing, 85
National Nurse Practitioner exam, 216
National Nurse Practitioner Residency Training Consortium, 218–219
National Organization of Nurse Practitioner Faculty (NONPF), 30–31, 50, 69, 86, 89, 95
  NP role core competencies, 51–52

The National Simulation Study, 68
National Task Force for Quality Nurse Practitioner Education, 69
navigating simulation, 78–81
  classification of simulation, 78
  simulation modalities, 79–81
Nesbit, 123
Netherlands
  APNs, 16–17
  certified nurse specialist (CNS), 16
  NPs, 17
networks, 206
Nicosia, F. M., 129
Nightengale, Florence, 63–64
NONPF guidelines, 95
No Surprises Act, 165
Nurse and Midwifery Board of Ireland, 17
Nurse Educator Core Competencies, 34–35
nurse educators, 34–35
nurse executive doctors of nursing practice (DNP), 35–36
nurse executives (NE), 35–36
nurse practice acts (NPAs), 198–199
nurse practitioners (NPs), 5, 8, 20
  Australia, 13–14
  Canada, 14–15
  clinical role of, 33–34
  international practice, 12–20
  Netherlands, 16
  nurse executive leadership, 35–36
  nursing informatics, 36–37
  specialty advanced practice roles, 34–40
  specialty certification, 33
  United Kingdom, 18–19
Nurses Improve Care for Health Systems Elders (NICHE), 113
nursing informatics, 36–37
nursing regulatory bodies (NRB), 198

O

Obama, Barack, 172
objective structured clinical examinations (OSCEs), 71
Olshansky, E. F., 217
Ortiz, J., 115

P

patient-centered care, 224–226
  principles of, 225
Patient Protection and Affordable Care Act (PPACA), 172
patient safety and appropriate use of telehealth, 127
People's Daily, 16
performance domains, 148–155
personal, professional, and leadership development, 204
person-centered care, 202, 224
Peterson, P. A., 206–207
physical safety, 82
physician assistants (PAs), 219
planning performance, 151–152, 155
PMI Code of Ethics and Professional Conduct, 147
Poghosyan, L., 207
policy, defined, 162
population health, 202–203
Poronsky, C. B., 217
post-simulation debriefing, 90
Practice Transition Accreditation Program (PTAP), 220
prebriefing
  as simulation phase, 86–89
  briefing, 86–87
  preparation, 86–89
Pregnancy Assistance Fund Program (PAFP), 178
Prelicensure Nursing Programs, 68–69
preparation, and prebriefing, 86–89
professionalism, 204
professional leadership, 142
Project Extension for Community Health care Outcomes (ECHO), 129
Project Management Institute, 156
project management (PM)
  defined, 146–147
  delivery performance, 152–153, 155
  development approach, 151, 155
  foundational principles, 147–148
  life cycle performance, 151, 155
  measurement performance, 153–155
  performance domains, 148–155

planning performance, 151–152, 155
project work performance, 152, 155
stakeholder performance, 150, 155
team performance, 150, 155
uncertainty performance, 154–155
project work performance, 152, 155
protected health information, 166
psychological safety, 82
Public Health and Social Services Emergency Fund, 183
Public Health Service Act (PHSA), 172
pyramid of professional competence, 75

Q

Qualified Clinical Data Registry (QCDR), 182
quality and safety, 203
quality improvement (QI), 142–143

R

real-time telemedicine, 126
reduced practice authority, 8, 10
the reflective practitioner theory, 74–75
registered nurse (RN), 198–199
licensure, 200
transition to advanced practice nurse, 215–227
reimbursement policies, 131–135
remote monitoring, 126–127
Republic of Ireland, 17–18
restricted practice, 9–10
Reynolds, Kim, 169–170
rural health care, 168
rural health care, and SDOHs, 115
Rural Hospital Transformation Act, 168

S

Sawatzky, J., 217
scholarship for nursing practice, 203
Schön, Donald A., 74, 89
Schubert, C., 70
self-confidence, 218
Sheer, Barbara, 4
Sichuan Provincial People's Hospital (SPPH), 16
Silver, Henry K., 3
"simulated participant" (SP), 81–83
simulation
benefits and limitations of, 75–77
classification of, 78
defined, 60
designing, 84–86
enhancing education and practice, 67–73
evaluation in, 92–94
evaluation tools, 94
evolution in, 63–67
formative evaluation, 92–93
high-stakes evaluation, 93–94
historical foundations of, 61–63
in advanced practice nursing, 59–97
in advanced practice nursing education, 94–95
methods of conducting, 83–84
modalities, 79–81
navigating, 78–81
overview, 60–61
"simulated participant" (SP), 81–83
summative evaluation, 93
simulation-based education (SBE), 61
simulation-based experiences (SBE), 85–87, 89, 92, 95–96
simulation delivery methods, 83–84
simulation design, 89
simulation phases, 86–92
debriefing, 89–92
prebriefing, 86–89
simulation design, 89
social care, 110–111
social determinants of health (SDOHs), 104–106
impacts on mental health, 114–115
impacts on rural health care, 115
social disadvantage, 109
social learning theory, 75
Social Security Amendments of 1965, 2
Spanish influenza pandemic of 1918–1919, 5
Special Supplemental Nutrition Program for Women, Infants, and Children (WIC), 182
stakeholder performance, 150, 155
state licensure, 200

St-Martin, L., 218, 220
"store-and-forward" technology, 126
student registered nurse anesthetist (SRNA), 39
summary of benefits and coverage (SBC), 175–176
summative evaluation, 93
systems-based practice, 203
systems leadership, 142

T

team adaptability, 63
team leader, 145
team performance, 150, 155
team strategies and tools to enhance performance and patient safety (Team STEPPS), 72
technology
  for telehealth, 127
  videoconferencing, 124, 126
telehealth, 11
  access in, 127
  advantages of, 128–130
  communication via, 127
  data collection and assessment via, 127
  defining, 122–124
  disadvantages of, 130
  equity in, 127
  ethical practices and legal requirements for, 128
  evolution of, 125
  patient safety and appropriate use of, 127
  technology for, 127
  types of, 126–127
telehealth competencies, 127–128
  access and equity in telehealth, 127
  communication via telehealth, 127
  data collection and assessment via telehealth, 127
  ethical practices/legal requirements for telehealth, 128
  patient safety and appropriate use of telehealth, 127
  technology for telehealth, 127
telemedicine
  asynchronous, 126
  defined, 122
  defining, 122–124
  mobile health (mHealth), 126
  real-time, 126
  remote monitoring, 126–127
  types of, 126–127
telepsychiatry, 11
theoretical frameworks, 73–75
  Knowles' adult learning theory, 74–75
  Kolb's experiential learning theory, 73–74
  the reflective practitioner theory, 74–75
To Err is Human: Building a Safer Health System, 65
tools to measure readiness for change, 144
transition from registered nurse to advanced practice nurse, 215–227
  communication, 222–224
  functioning as member of the health care team, 224
  overview, 216–221
  patient-centered care, 224–226
  role transition, 221–222
transition-to-practice (TTP) programs, 219
Trump administration, 167

U

uncertainty performance, 154–155
undergraduate nursing education, 68
United Kingdom
  NPs, 19
United States, levels of supervision, 205–208
U.S. Department of Agriculture (USDA), 182
U.S. Preventive Services Task Force (USPSTF), 176

V

Veterans Administration TeleSleep program, 129
videoconferencing technology, 124, 126
virtual check-ins, 132
virtual reality (VR), 124
virtual visits, 132
vulnerability, defined, 107

vulnerable populations, 107–108
  advanced practice role in caring for, 113–114

W
Ward, Lillian, 5
Wilson, E., 21
Women's Health Nurse Practitioners (WHNP), 37
Wood, E., 40
World Health Organization (WHO), 6–8, 34
World War I, 5–6
World War II, 6, 65

ABOUT THE EDITOR

Dr. Carole Mackavey, DNP, MSN, APRN, FNP-C is an associate professor at the Cizik School of Nursing/University of Texas Health Science Center in Houston, Texas. She is the MSN program coordinator and the post masters nursing education track coordinator. She primarily teaches in the BSN to DNP and MSN nursing education programs. A native of Newton, Massachusetts, Dr. Mackavey moved to Texas in 1998 and attended the University of Texas Medical Branch at Galveston, where she earned a Master of Science in Nursing/FNP. After many years of practicing in the Heights area as a family nurse practitioner, she earned a Doctor of Nursing Practice degree at UTHealth. Dr. Mackavey has been actively involved in advanced nursing practice education for 18 years. Her areas of interest are the advanced practice nurse role development in the U.S. and abroad, and competency-based education. She often uses gamification strategies to enhance student engagement and stimulate critical thinking, uses simulation modalities to improve clinical knowledge and skill proficiency, and develops curriculum and measurement approaches for advanced nurse practice education.

ABOUT THE CONTRIBUTORS

Dr. Linda Cole, DNP, RN, CCNS, CNE, FCNS Dr. Cole, associate professor at the Cizik School of Nursing (CSON) at the University of Texas Health Science Center, Houston, teaches various courses in the master's-level Nursing Leadership and DNP programs and holds leadership responsibilities in the MSN programs. Her BSN and MS in health education are from the University of Southern Mississippi in Hattiesburg, MS, and her MSN as a clinical nurse specialist and DNP are from CSON. Dr. Cole was inducted as a Clinical Nurse Specialist Institute Fellow in 2021. She has published and presented on evidence-based practice, integrative medicine, nursing leadership, and nurse resiliency.

Dr. Mandi Lyons, DNP, APRN, WHNP-BC, CHSE Dr. Mandi Lyons is an assistant professor and the co-director of simulation at Cizik School of Nursing. She obtained her advanced practice nursing degree and Doctor of Nursing Practice at the Cizik School of Nursing. She specializes in reproductive health care and health care simulation and has utilized simulated experiences for future nurses and nurse practitioners to practice the application of theory for the health and care of women, newborns, and families. She has 20 years of experience working with underserved populations as a registered nurse (RN) and a women's health nurse practitioner (WHNP). In addition to her clinical experience, Dr. Lyons is a certified health care simulation expert with over 5 years of health care simulation development, application, and evaluation experience in undergraduate, graduate, and interprofessional courses. Her goal in health care education is to expand on the current knowledge of simulation and "gamification" within health care education settings as well as develop interactive and realistic learning environments. She has also worked as a consultant for companies such as Shadow Health (2021) Virtual Simulation Program (bought by Elsevier) and Elsevier's Simulation Learning System (current), refining their globally used simulation content. In her spare time, she spends time with her two children, ages 8 and 2, and enjoys reading psychological thrillers, playing video games and board games, and crafting with her Cricut.

Padmavathy Ramaswamy, PhD, MPH, APRN, FNP-BC Dr. Padmavathy Ramaswamy is an assistant professor at the Cizik School of Nursing at the University of Texas Health Science Center in Houston. She is a university-wide Interprofessional Education (IPE) Executive Council member. She actively coordinates and leads multiple IPE activities as a member of the university's Center of Interprofessional Collaboration and is a noted speaker on IPE.

Her doctoral research focused on the use of mobile health (mHealth) technology among South Asians living in the United States. Her research interest focuses on the use of mHealth and other technologies aimed at health promotion and disease prevention, especially among older adults.

She has earned multiple degrees, including a PhD in nursing, an MPH, an MSN, and post-master's certificates in applied health informatics and nursing education. Her 20-year clinical experience as a family nurse practitioner spans the population and age spectrum. She maintains an active faculty clinical practice at the University of Houston Student Health Center.

Lisa Boss, PhD, EdD, RN, CNS, CEN, CNE Dr. Lisa Boss is assistant dean for curriculum and instruction and associate professor of the tenure track at Tarleton State University in Stephenville, Texas. Dr. Boss primarily teaches in the Master of Science in

Nursing program in the Nursing Administration and Nursing Education tracks, where her expertise in nursing education and leadership are best applied. Dr. Boss began her educational journey in 1997 and obtained educational degrees at the University of Texas Medical Branch in Galveston (BSN), the University of Texas Health Science Center at Houston (MSN, post-master's, and PhD), and the University of Houston (EdD). Dr. Boss's research in nursing education is related to simulation and leadership, and her research in patient health outcomes is biobehavioral with a focus on various vulnerable populations, psychosocial and biological factors, and how these factors impact health outcomes.

Kelly Kearney, DNP, APRN, PMHNP-BC Dr. Kearney is an associate professor and director of the PMHNP program at Cizik School of Nursing at the University of Texas Health Science Center in Houston. She has worked as a psychiatric mental health nurse Practitioner (PMHNP) for the past 11 years. Much of that time has been spent in outpatient psychiatry, treating children, adolescents, and adults with various mental health disorders. Dr. Kearney serves on the Board of Directors for Ronald McDonald House Charities of the Greater Houston/Galveston area as the vice president of programming. She is the regional representative for the Psychiatric Advanced Practice Nurses of Texas. Additionally, she is a National Organization of Nurse Practitioner Faculties member and holds a 2-year appointment to the diversity committee. Other national committees of which she is a member include the International Society for Psychiatric-Mental Health Nurses, the American Psychiatric Nurses Association, and Sigma Theta Tau International Honor Society of Nurses.

Dr. Kearney's research areas are psychiatry, diversity, equity, inclusion (DEI), and graduate education. She is a co-investigator of a 2.6-million-dollar grant (Advanced Nursing Education Workforce) funded by HRSA. She previously was a co-investigator for the Workplace Violence Prevention grant in collaboration with Harris County Psychiatric Center.

Kathleen Siders, DNP, MSN, APRN, FNP-C Kathleen Siders is an assistant professor at Cizik School of Nursing and has 49 years of experience as a registered nurse, serving as a family nurse practitioner for the past 20 years. She has been faculty in the Graduate Studies Department at Cizik School of Nursing with UTHealth-Houston since 2014. She has served in leadership positions with the director of the BSN-to-DNP program since 2018. Her interests include teaching clinical reasoning and structuring faculty–student advisement.

Robert Coghlan, PhD, RN, MA, MSN, CNS, FNP Dr. Robert Coghlan has been involved in health care for nearly 40 years. His interest in health policy led him to the University of Houston, where he earned his PhD in political science, studying the fields of policy sciences, methodology, and American government. He completed his dissertation, "The Influence of the Media in Healthcare Reform," in 2011.

Dr. Coghlan has had an extensive career in health care leadership, in hospitals and the private sector. His most recent leadership role was as chief operating officer and chief nursing officer, leading two emergency hospitals. He also assisted in developing three different electronic medical records, led the Forms Committee, reviewed and updated hospital- and corporate-wide policies, developed new service lines, and mentored others.

Dr. Aastha Krebs, DNP, MBA-HCM, PMHNP-BC Dr. Aastha Krebs is a psychiatric mental health nurse practitioner specializing in mental health advocacy and policy research. Currently serving at Whitman-Walker Health, a Federally Qualified Health Center (FQHC) in Washington, DC, she is dedicated to enhancing access to mental health care, reducing stigma, and promoting health care equity through a combination of clinical expertise, education, and advocacy for health policy. Aastha earned her Doctor of Nursing Practice degree from the University of Texas Health Science Center at Houston and holds a Master of Business Administration in Healthcare Management from Western Governors University.

Tammy L. Stout, DNP, APRN, ACNP-BC Dr. Stout is an assistant professor program director for the Adult-Gerontology Acute Care Nurse Practitioner program at the University of Texas Health Science Center Cizik School of Nursing. She began her career as a licensed vocational nurse. She went on to obtain a Bachelor of Science in Nursing (1987); a master's in nursing science as an acute care nurse practitioner (2001); and, finally, her Doctor of Nursing Practice degree (2011). Her areas of interest are cardiopulmonary medicine with a focus on clinical and hospital medicine, internal medicine, hospice, and palliative care. She has held multiple leadership positions, including director of clinical nursing, director of advanced nursing for Harbor HealthCare Systems, and chief operations officer for Tri-Met Medical Services PA.

www.ingramcontent.com/pod-product-compliance
Ingram Content Group UK Ltd.
Pitfield, Milton Keynes, MK11 3LW, UK
UKHW021831270726
14058UKWH00001B/88